The Jack Sprat Low-Fat Diet

THE
Jack Sprat
LOW-FAT DIET

A 28-DAY HEART-HEALTHY PLAN
YOU CAN FOLLOW
THE REST OF YOUR LIFE

Dr. Bryant A. Stamford and Becca Coffin, R.N.

THE UNIVERSITY PRESS OF KENTUCKY

Scholarly publisher for the Commonwealth,
serving Bellarmine College, Berea College, Centre
College of Kentucky, Eastern Kentucky University,
The Filson Club, Georgetown College, Kentucky
Historical Society, Kentucky State University,
Morehead State University, Murray State University,
Northern Kentucky University, Transylvania University,
University of Kentucky, University of Louisville,
and Western Kentucky University.

Editorial and Sales Offices: The University Press of Kentucky
663 South Limestone Street, Lexington, Kentucky 40508-4008

Library of Congress Cataloging-in-Publication Data

Stamford, Bryant A.
    The Jack Sprat low-fat diet : a 28-day heart-healthy plan you can
follow the rest of your life / Bryant A. Stamford and Becca Coffin.
        p.   cm.
    Includes bibliographical references and index.
    ISBN 0–8131–0856–X (alk. paper)
    1. Low-fat diet—Recipes.   I. Coffin, Becca, 1948–
II. Title.
RM237.7.S76   1995
613.2′8—dc20   95–24064

Contents

Part Three On Your Own

Prologue
The Legacy of Jack Sprat

Jack Sprat could eat no fat
His wife could eat no lean
And so between them both, you see
They licked the platter clean
　　—In John Clark, *Paroemiologia Anglo-Latina,* 1639

Sounds like a pretty good relationship—perfect compatibility. And it was. Jack loved his wife dearly, and their love thrived for many years, even though Mrs. Sprat grew in size while Jack stayed slender and handsome.

Jack never said a word to his wife about her weight, not wanting to upset her. But he worried about her health, especially when Mrs. Sprat began to show signs that all was not right inside her body. She fatigued easily, breaking out in a deep sweat at the slightest exertion, and she complained of feeling out-of-sorts and of not being able to sleep well.

Jack was convinced his wife's problems were caused by her weight. But he was at a loss to understand why she weighed so much. They ate together at every meal; he ate much more food than she did, and, until recently, they had worked side by side in the fields from dawn to dusk. Her weight problem was a real mystery to Jack.

One evening after a large meal, Mrs. Sprat told Jack she was having chest pains. Jack knew this could be trouble, and he was off immediately to fetch the doctor. But when they returned, they found Mrs. Sprat dead in her bed. Heart attack, the doctor said.

Jack was very sad, especially at the dinner table, because he had no one to eat the fat. He thought that maybe he should eat the fat himself—waste not, want not. But he couldn't.

Eventually, Jack married again. The new Mrs. Sprat loved to eat fat even more than his first wife, and mealtime was just as it had been in the old days. But she grew to be immense, and tragedy struck again. This time it was colon cancer, the doctor said.

Jack married four more times, each marriage a model of compatibility. His wives ate the fat; he ate the lean. But each marriage ended tragically. Jack buried his sixth wife when he was ninety-three. She was decades younger. Alas, all of his wives had died big and fat and at a young age. Depressed, Jack vowed never to marry again—the pain of losing six wives was too much for him.

Jack spent the next twenty years confused and lonely, and wondering why he had had such bad luck with his wives. Then one day as he was out walking after dinner, he came upon the town wizard, who stood on a tree stump, busily instructing his apprentices on healthful eating. Jack crept behind a bush and listened as the wizard raised his voice and waved his arms about, condemning the evils of dietary fat and its health-destroying ways.

Aha! Jack thought. This was the answer he had been seeking for twenty years. Eating fat was the reason for the heart disease, colon cancer, diabetes, high blood pressure, and gallbladder attacks his wives had suffered. Eating fat was the reason his wives were obese and had died before their times. Oh, how he wished he had known this many years before.

Having solved the mystery, Jack revoked his vow and decided to search for a new wife. Although he was one hundred thirteen years old, he was still slender and handsome and full of vitality. Soon he met a charming young woman, Helga, and fell head-over-heels in love. But there was a problem. Helga loved to eat fat. Jack was disappointed and didn't know what to do, so he went to the town wizard for advice.

"Here is what you must do," the wizard told Jack. "Ask Helga to eat the lean for just one month. And tell her that if she chooses to go back to her old ways when the month is up, you will allow it and you will never question her choice."

"But—" cried Jack, fearful that the plan might fail. "What if—"

The wizard raised his hand, silencing Jack. "Trust in the power of the lean. It has served you well all these many years, and it will not let you down now."

Jack was skeptical, but he decided to give the wizard's advice a try. Helga listened attentively as Jack explained the plan. She was reluctant—she had never eaten the lean before—but her love for Jack was strong, and finally she agreed. At first, meals were grim affairs. Helga would frown and push the food Jack had prepared around her plate with her fork, looking for fat that wasn't there. But, true to her word, she ate the lean, and each day she ate a little more. Gradually, her frown disappeared.

The days went by, and Helga found that the more lean she ate, the more she liked it. Soon she was eating as much as Jack. Then something wonderful happened. After supper on the twenty-eighth day, Helga turned to Jack and said, "I have never felt better in my life. I will never go back to eating the fat."

Jack was so happy, he married Helga the very next day. They lived happily—and healthfully—ever after.

Introduction
Pocket Full of Miracles

Jack Sprat ate more food than his wives—a whole lot more. He and his wives worked side by side in the fields from dawn to dusk, but Jack remained slim while his wives became obese, and Jack stayed healthy and vital whereas his wives died prematurely.

Is there a mystery here?

Not really, not once you understand the modus operandi of dietary fat. Fat is sinister. Like an addictive narcotic, it pulls you in and captures your taste buds. It tastes heavenly on the way in, but once inside, it wreaks havoc on every system of the body. Eating fat makes you fat, but that's just the beginning. It clogs your arteries, raises your blood pressure, overloads your bowels, and gives you diabetes. And, of course, when it's done with you, it kills you.

Dietary fat is a cold-blooded mass murderer, and it must be stopped. Fortunately, this message is beginning to sink into the American psyche. That's the good news. The bad news is it will be years before a real impact is felt.

The battle against cigarette smoking is a useful example. Three decades ago, the health-destroying power of cigarette smoking was becoming apparent. Millions of puffers took note, and they began talking about it. "I probably ought to quit," some would say, as they lit another cigarette. Eventually, the "I ought to quit" thinking took hold, and our society underwent a tremendous shift in consciousness to the point that today, cigarette smokers are a dwindling minority.

Just as we began to recognize the dangers of cigarette smoking thirty years ago, we are beginning to recognize today that dietary fat is bad for us, and we are beginning to talk about it. We stuff ourselves with sludge-filled bacon cheeseburgers and 12-ounce servings of prime rib, then wink and say, "I probably shouldn't be eating this." Talking doesn't accomplish much, but it's a first step. This book was written to help you take additional steps.

When you accept the fact that fat is evil, the next step is to take action. Unfortunately, your good intentions may set you up for a fall. Unscrupulous food producers, who know that a growing segment of the American public wants to lower their dietary fat intake, can manipulate your good intentions. Instead of changing their products and lowering the fat content, many companies simply alter their advertising claims. Your eagerness to change also may cause you to fall victim to the latest flimflam diet. Or you may make honest mistakes, caused by naïveté and lack of knowledge. You may think you are doing better than you really are. Meanwhile, precious time is wasted, and you keep gaining fat and losing health.

This book will provide everything you need to know to guide you through the jungle of deceit. The chapters are short and to the point. We offer a simplified text that distills the facts to bare-bones accounts and requires minimal reading time.

In part 1 we will prepare you for the Jack Sprat diet plan. It is important that you read the chapters carefully *before* starting the plan. Your success depends not only on commitment and determination but also on a firm understanding of *why* you are doing what you are doing. Every step must make sense to you, and every step must be appreciated for its role in contributing to overall success.

In part 2 you will begin active participation in the 28-day plan. We will walk you through, step by step. The resources contain recipes used in the 28-day menus and other valuable information necessary for you to carry out the plan successfully.

After you get started on the plan and feel comfortable, you will want to read part 3. It will expand your understanding of body fat, healthy eating, and exercise. We firmly believe that, in the long run, the more you know, the more success you will enjoy and sustain.

The Jack Sprat diet plan is practical and based in reality. It is effective, and it will feel comfortably familiar right from the beginning. We have included fast foods and have even incorporated a system of "controlled cheating." Because many of the foods you will be eating will be familiar, you won't feel like you are on a diet. That's precisely what we had in mind. You will change your eating habits, but you won't notice that much difference. Your body will notice a big difference, however, and it will thank you by becoming healthier and losing fat.

We offer no fancy high-tech breakthroughs to speed you along. There is no "correct" combination of food enzymes that will melt blubber from your waistline. There is no transistorized gadget to emulsify cellulite from your thighs. There is only common sense and know-how. You supply the common sense, and we'll give you the know-how. The best thing about what we have to offer is that, once adopted, the Jack Sprat plan will serve you for the rest of your life.

The plan uses a guided "spoon-fed" approach that has been individualized as much as possible with regard to gender, size, and physical activity level. A special feature of the plan is that it is both a weight-loss and a weight-maintenance program. How is that possible? We'll tell you later. For now, all you need to know is that once you reach your desired (target) weight, there is no need to change a thing. This innovative approach provides you the comfort of knowing that once you adapt to the 28-day plan, no further changes are necessary.

Each of the four weeks in the plan starts with a complete grocery list. Ours is not the generic grocery list you've seen in diet plans that are nothing more than pages of tables. Take our list to the market, follow it from beginning to end, checking off items as you go, and you will have everything you need for the week's menus. The menus for each day have been analyzed to let you know, item by item, how many calories and grams of fat and saturated fat you will be consuming. Recipes are included for each of the home-prepared items that appear in the 28-day plan.

We are aware that not everyone will like our food selections. Not to worry. Our series of specially designed substitution tables will help you. If you don't care for a particular food—the main course for lunch on Day 2 of the week, for example—all you have to do is consult the tables and choose a substitute with approximately the same number of calories and fat grams. Recipes are included for all selections in the tables. This approach adds flexibility while ensuring the consistency of the plan.

Although we feel strongly that you will benefit from 28 days on the plan, we realize that it may not be feasible for everyone. Strange working hours, uncooperative family members, and other problems may make commitment to the plan impossible. So be it. You may, however, be able to follow the plan in a spotty fashion a day or two a week. This is not ideal, of course, but each day you are on the plan, the experience you receive will teach you something valuable. This, added to what you will have learned from reading the chapters in this book, will enable you to make smart choices in the future that will benefit you greatly.

The goal of the Jack Sprat diet plan is to reduce your fat intake to not more than 20 percent of total calories, with as little saturated fat as possible. The daily menus range from 10 to 20 percent fat, with an average of 15 percent. In our experience, this level of fat intake results in the substantial loss of body fat—even without cutting calories—and a dramatic change in one's health profile (serum cholesterol, blood pressure, and so forth). It is also a level of fat intake that allows sufficient variety in the diet to keep meals interesting. You won't be limited to rabbit food, in other words.

Why 28 days?

We created the plan as a means to introduce you to low-fat "smart" eating, and then to solidify your commitment.

When you complete the 28 days, will you go back to your old habits?

No way! Once you've conditioned your taste buds to smart eating, they won't allow you to go back. If you give up drinking whole milk, you may find, at first, that 2 percent milk tastes hollow, but eventually you will get used to it. Then if you switch to 1 percent, it may taste like dishwater at first, but gradually your taste buds will grow to like it. Finally, if you take the big plunge to skim, you will adjust to that too. Once you've grown fond of skim milk, whole milk will taste bad to you.

Just give yourself a chance, and you will be amazed at how much and how quickly you can change.

Should you expect miracles?

That depends. If you expect to become trim and beautiful in 28 days, we can't help you. No one can, regardless of their claims. But if your expectations are a little lower, we can provide you a whole pocket full of miracles: (1) you will be eating more food than ever before, and the food will be tasty and satisfying; (2) you will experience painless and comfortable weight loss, and you will keep the weight off; (3) you will have more energy than you thought possible; and (4) you will look and feel better than you have in years.

Will you become bored and tempted to bolt from the plan?

Not at all. There is plenty of variety in this plan to keep you happy. The average person repeats food selections within a 28-day cycle, often several times, without feeling bored or confined. Therefore, the Jack Sprat 28-day diet plan probably contains more variety than you are used to. What's more, you are not limited to 28 days of selections. When you want to try something new and different, all you need to do is consult the substitution tables. And if you uncover an unusual concoction in a magazine or elsewhere that looks promising, simply determine the caloric content and the fat grams, then substitute it into the plan. We'll show you how.

What if you have a Big Mac attack?

No problem. We've got you covered. Controlled cheating on the plan offers four "warthog" days from which to choose. You will have your choice of pizza, fried chicken, Mexican food, or a big burger and fries. No one's perfect, and at some point in the 28-day plan you may encounter a powerful urge. Simply page ahead to the warthog section, pick one of the days, and go for it. The important thing is that you operate within the plan—even when you cheat. As satisfying as a warthog day may be, you will still be well below your normal fat intake.

When you complete 28 days, you will have a number of options. One is to repeat the cycle, again and again. Two is to repeat the cycle, but with adjustments you've made (and may continue to make) that make the plan more personalized and more palatable. Three is to "graduate" from the structure of the plan and forge ahead on your own, using what you've learned, and picking and choosing from the plan and the substitution tables to make a new system just for you.

Whatever you decide, we are confident you will never go

back to your old ways of eating. You may not be perfect, but you will be a whole lot better off than you were before.

We would wish you luck, but you won't need it. Simply follow Jack Sprat's lead, and everything will take care of itself.

Part One
Prepping for the Plan

I

Dumping the Diet Mentality

The Jack Sprat plan is a first step toward permanent change. It is a means to an end, in other words, and not an end in itself. This fact alone makes it unique. When people enter into crash diets, they do so with the understanding that they will be on the diet for only a short while. The shortness allows them to endure, encourages them to continue in the face of extreme discomfort.

The folly of this line of thinking is obvious. Abandon the changes you've made and the weight comes back. This is why the vast majority of diets fail in the short run, and virtually all diets fail in the long run. More on this in the next chapter.

When we started putting together the Jack Sprat plan, we wanted to expand the emphasis beyond weight loss. This, we hoped would create a different mind-set, one that was not driven by unrealistic expectations and obsessed with lower numbers on the scale. We hoped it would increase the likelihood that new eating habits would develop and be sustained. We knew that once new habits were adopted, positive changes would follow.

We also understand and respect the power of old habits, especially those you have nurtured from the cradle. If you are thirty years old, you have a thirty-year eating habit to contend with. If you are fifty, it's worse, because the longer the habit, the stronger the habit. But it's possible, and it can happen in only 28 days.

You will lose weight. Guaranteed. More important, you will lose body fat, and each pound of lost body fat will noticeably improve your appearance. Most dieters have never had this experience because on crash diets you lose mostly muscle and water.

Here are two examples of what can happen if you make smart choices, eat to be healthy, and quit worrying about weight loss.

The Becca Coffin Story

My father became very ill when I was a teenager, suffering with stomach ulcers and heart disease. On doctor's advice, he changed his eating habits, mostly limiting his intake of fried and spicy foods to keep his ulcer from acting up. Little was known about the heart disease–dietary fat link at the time. In fact, I remember fixing my father milk shakes with ice cream, whole milk, and eggs—foods that were supposed to soothe his ulcer. These same foods, unfortunately, were loaded with artery-clogging saturated fat.

I wish we had known then what we know now. Eating right and making smart choices will extend life and ensure quality of life in the later years. My father was willing to change his eating habits. He showed this. But he just didn't know how to do it right. He died from a heart attack at age sixty-two.

Despite my father's problems, I felt smug about my health. I didn't smoke or drink and was fairly active. I believed I was "eating right" too, with the exception of fast-food lunches and my need for peanut M&Ms. The fact is, when I looked around at what my friends were eating, I believed my eating habits were pretty good. I could even rationalize my pizzas, having learned in nursing school that pizza was a good source of nutrition, and protein especially. What I didn't realize was how much fat was in the pizza, the fast foods, and the M&M's.

Over the years I had put on a few extra pounds, but didn't everybody? I wished those pounds weren't there, but I wasn't prepared to run marathons to get rid of them.

In my forties, I started working with Dr. Stamford at the Health Promotion Center at the University of Louisville. It didn't take me long to learn that I wasn't the epitome of health I had imagined I was. My serum cholesterol, I learned, was 245 mg/dl. That's well above average, and much too high. It scared me. Here I was approaching middle age and menopause, a time when a woman's risk of heart disease increases dramatically. I needed to make changes, or risk sharing my father's fate.

The Jack Sprat eating plan came to the rescue. I became aware of just how much fat I had been consuming with my less than careful eating. It was astonishing. About three months after starting the Jack Sprat plan, I had my serum cholesterol tested again. It had dropped more than 40 points. Today, I keep it down in the 180s.

I had expected my cholesterol to drop because I cut the saturated fat from my diet. But I was eating a lot of food, and I didn't expect to lose weight. It just sort of "happened."

Overall, I lost fifteen pounds! (That's a lot when you are only a little over five feet tall.) Old clothes that were a little too tight now hung on my hips. I even felt comfortable wearing a two-piece bathing suit again, because there was no excess fat hanging around my midsection.

I don't want to give you the idea that this was the first time I had ever lost weight. It wasn't. I've tried my share of crash diets, especially in my younger days, and the weight came off. But I could never continue the drastic changes the diets required, and the weight came right back on. Now I know, of course, that the weight I had lost on these crazy diets wasn't fat but muscle and water, and that's why I gained it back. I know the weight I've lost on the Jack Sprat plan is fat. And I know it won't come back. It's been gone for years.

The Bryant Stamford Story

Years ago I was an exercise fanatic, posting big mileage on the jogging trail. I assumed I was healthy as a horse and paid no attention whatsoever to my eating habits. Why should I? My body was like a blast furnace, quickly burning off everything that entered.

The only blemish on my physique was a set of stubborn love handles—deposits of fat at my sides just above the beltline. The handles were leftovers from my power-lifting bulk-up days in my twenties when I was forty pounds heavier. I hated those handles, but no amount of side bends, sit-ups, or running mileage would get rid of them.

For years I assumed my love handles were my only major (bodily) defect. Then I had my cholesterol tested. It was 210 mg/dl. That's about average for American adults. But I never thought of myself as average. Indeed I wasn't, I came to learn. My HDL—the good type of cholesterol that helps keep the arteries clean, was frightfully low, a genetic condition. This gave me an unhealthy ratio (total cholesterol divided by HDL) of 6.2 to 1. Average for American men is 5 to 1. I was worse than average, which meant my risk of heart disease was higher.

Panicked, I decided to exercise more, doubling my mileage. This shows how little I understood the issues at the time. All that running made me more fit—as fit as I had ever been in my life—but it didn't solve my problem. My cholesterol stayed high, my HDL stayed low, and my love handles stayed put.

Desperate, I decided to take a look at my diet. It was horrible. My daily lunches at McDonald's supplied more than 1,200 calories and 74 grams of fat. My meaty dinners were no healthier, and it was not uncommon for me to have eggs and bacon or sausage for breakfast. No wonder my cholesterol was a mess. My arteries cringe at the memory.

I needed to change, and change fast. I quit fast-food lunches in favor of things like tuna packed in spring water. This change alone made a dramatic impact on my cholesterol. Bolstered by my success, I switched to oatmeal for breakfast and broiled fish for dinner. My cholesterol kept dropping, all the way to 140 mg/dl.

I found that the more lean I ate, the more I liked it. I began "grazing"—chewing on whole grain breads and rolls and fruits and vegetable sticks throughout the day. I was eating more than ever, but I didn't feel stuffed and lazy. I snacked too, but on low-fat items. My cholesterol dropped further, to the 120 range, a level common among vegetarians. The average person doesn't need to go this low. Certainly, I didn't try. It just happened because I was eating right.

With all my attention focused on cholesterol, I didn't pay much attention to my physique. My belt had come in a few notches, and my weight was down about ten pounds, but I didn't think much about it because the change was gradual. Then one day I was cleaning out a closet and found a pair of swimming trunks. They looked like new, and the tag was still attached. Then I remembered. I had bought them a few years before, but banished them because the elastic waist band squeezed under my love handles, thrusting them up and out like a push-up bra. Ugh!

I slipped on the trunks and went to the mirror. The love handles were hardly noticeable. I flexed my abdominal muscles and found the outline was sharper than it had been in years, even though I had quit punishing myself with countless sit-ups and leg lifts.

The common thread running through our stories and those of many others is transformation without "dieting." The changes occurred simply because we began making smart choices.

2

Fool's Gold

"Crash diets are fool's gold: they promise much but provide nothing." This was Jack Sprat's response to anyone who suggested his wife should go on a diet to lose weight. There was no way he was going to urge his wife to deny herself good things to eat, to endure itsy-bitsy servings, and to torture herself with never-ending temptations, only to lose a few pounds that came right back on.

Jack was right. To be sure, you will lose weight on a diet, but most of the weight you lose won't be fat. It will be muscle and water. If you think the distinction is merely technical, you're wrong.

Lose fat, and you will look and feel great, and your health profile will improve dramatically. But none of these positive outcomes will occur without *fat* loss, no matter how many *pounds* you lose.

Body fat is extremely compact, squeezing a whopping 9 calories of energy into every gram. That adds up to 3,500 calories per pound of stored fat. Calling fat from storage is difficult. And even if you are successful in prying open the fat cell doors, the sheer magnitude of the number of calories that need to be expended to lose only one pound presents quite a challenge.

The first law of thermodynamics tells us that energy is neither created nor destroyed. It can be transferred, but it must always be accounted for; it cannot simply disappear. Body fat must be converted to usable energy, in other words, in order to make it disappear.

You can do this by dieting—consuming fewer calories (less energy), which means you are relying upon your existing fat stores to make up for the loss of energy intake. This sounds good, but according to the Set Point Theory, if you cut your caloric intake too drastically, your metabolic rate plummets in an attempt to protect your fat stores. Your body, unfortunately, assumes that when you cut calories, you are in the throes of a famine, and the longer your fat stores last, the longer you stay alive.

You also can convert body fat to energy through exercise.

A brisk one-mile walk expends about 100 calories (for a 180-pound person), or ⅓₅ of a pound. A runner burns less than 1 pound of fat during a 26-mile marathon.

With an energy capacity of 3,500 calories per pound, it doesn't take a rocket scientist to see that it's impossible to lose fat quickly by dieting and/or exercise. You simply cannot expend enough calories in a short period of time.

But don't despair. You will lose fat. The Jack Sprat plan will gradually deplete your fat stores at the rate of approximately 1 pound per week, depending upon your chosen level of physical activity. This is an optimal rate.

Hold on, you say. You know lots of people who have lost 10 or 15 pounds in the first few weeks on a crash diet. How is that possible?

It's easy. Too easy, unfortunately, and that's why crash diets are so popular. The immediate loss of pounds leads you to believe the crash diet is working. It excites you because you think you are really accomplishing something. Sorry. All you are doing is losing muscle and water, and the lost inches result from shrinkage of your cells as they dehydrate.

Crash diets work by putting your body in a state of semistarvation shock, usually through a reduction in carbohydrate intake. The body has a modest amount of carbohydrates stored in long chains of glucose called glycogen, but the supply doesn't last long. And since glycogen is stored with water at a ratio of approximately three parts water to one part glycogen, depletion of 1 pound of glycogen results in a quick 4-pound weight loss.

Depletion of glycogen means depletion of stored glucose. This creates a major problem, because glucose is an essential fuel for the brain and nervous system. Without glucose, your brain won't work! But your body is too smart to allow the brain to shut down, and it resorts to survival-mode tactics. You begin breaking down muscle proteins and converting them to a makeshift form of glucose. This solves the problem for a while, but in the process several pounds of muscle are lost.

No one goes on a diet to lose muscle. When you look in the bathroom mirror and see unwelcome bulges, you don't say to yourself: "I wish I could get rid of all that darned muscle." When your twenty-year high school reunion approaches, you don't fret that former classmates will make comments behind your back about the additional muscle you've acquired since graduation.

But crash diets cause you to lose muscle at a rapid rate. This is because muscle is mostly water and supplies only a handful of usable calories per pound. This means you can burn through many pounds of muscle in the time it would take you to shed just one pound of fat. Crash diet advocates know this, and that's why they always guarantee fast *weight* loss. They never guarantee fast *fat* loss, because that's impossible.

Early in a crash diet, approximately 70 percent of weight loss is muscle and water. Eventually, more fat will be lost (along with the muscle and water), but most people drop out well before any significant amount of fat is lost—because they look and feel so bad, they wish they were dead. The only thing that keeps you going in a crash diet is the lower number on the scale, and even that can't keep you going for long.

This underscores two primary characteristics of crash diets. One, they are short-lived. And two, no new lifestyle habits are developed.

As if a crash diet isn't bad enough, things get worse when you quit. When the diet is over, you quickly return to old eating habits. This creates another major problem, because while you are on the diet, your metabolic rate is depressed. Two factors are operating. One, you have lost muscle mass, and muscle drives your metabolic rate. And, two, when you lower your caloric intake radically, your metabolism drops in an effort to preserve stored energy—to keep you from starving to death. These two effects don't go away just because you quit the diet.

On the contrary, even though you return to your old, sludge-filled eating ways, your metabolism acts as if you are still on the diet. It's still slowed down, in other words, and because you have less muscle mass to burn calories, you get a double whammy. The result? Your weight comes back in a rush. But remember, you lost mostly muscle and water. The weight that returns is mostly fat. Thus, when you return to your former weight, you are fatter than you were before you started the diet. And if all of the muscle you lost returns, it will push you to a higher body weight. Now you are not only fatter, but you weigh more too. Losing then gaining, then losing and gaining again is the crash diet "yo-yo" effect you've heard of.

Hardly worth the effort, is it?

Unfortunately, the American approach to reducing body fat is the same one we apply to the national debt. We recognize the importance of reduction, but we refuse to take the challenging steps required to get the job done. Instead we opt for quick fixes. And because our approach is so inept, our stores of body fat keep getting larger. Despite Nutrasweet, fake fat, and fancy weight-loss programs, Americans are fatter than ever before.

We spend more than $10 billion annually on weight-loss programs that clearly don't work. But we keep pouring our hard-earned cash into crash weight-loss programs, hoping to find the right one. We won't find the right one because they are all more or less the same.

So how can you tell when you are being ripped off by the latest fad diet?

It's hard to know, but help may be on the way. New York City has recognized that many weight-loss programs are flim-flams and is trying to help citizens make better decisions by forcing programs to disclose success rates. This is a great idea, but we suspect that the success rates reported will be massaged so that they bear little resemblance to the truth. The weight-loss industry will try to kill this venture, of course, and will probably succeed.

For success rates to be meaningful, they must reflect long-term success. Knowing that you can lose 50 pounds in a program is not helpful if you gain back 60 pounds soon after the program ends. Even so, weight-loss advertisements tell you that you will lose 20, 30, or more pounds quickly. Never is there a mention of how successful you will be keeping it off. The reason is, odds are stacked against you at about 99 to 1 that you will be anywhere close to keeping off even a portion of your diet-induced loses one year later.

If weight-loss programs insist on reporting short-term results, they should be required to determine and reveal what proportion of the weight loss was body fat and what proportion was muscle and water. If the weight loss was broken down into its components, you could compute an eye-opening net score that would show just how foolish rapid weight loss is.

To compute the net score, you subtract the number of pounds of lost muscle and water from the number of pounds of lost fat. For example, if you lost 50 pounds, but 25 was muscle and water and 25 pounds was fat, the score would be zero. In most cases, the score would be a negative number because on crash diets you lose more muscle and water than fat. This helps put a 50-pound weight loss in perspective.

Fortunately, after reading this book, you won't need a New York City law to protect you from crash diet scams. You will be a well-educated consumer who won't fall for tantalizing, but misleading, advertisements.

Recent medical studies have examined the success of expensive liquid diets. Most liquid diet programs are sponsored by hospitals or medical clinics. They cost more than $100 per week, they last about 26 weeks, and they usually begin with liquid-only meals, which provide 400-800 calories daily. This is a concentration camp ration, guaranteed to help you lose lots of muscle and water quickly.

Participants slowly graduate to eating food again, at which time the caloric content is increased to 1,000-1,500 calories a day. This is still too few calories for a large person, and the loss of muscle and water continues, but at a reduced rate.

One research study followed 517 individuals who entered a liquid diet program. Of the 285 who finished and were questioned one year later, only 24 hadn't gained back any weight.

We know at least a dozen or so individuals who have completed liquid diet programs. We also know a large number of dropouts. Of those who completed the program, all of them lost a great deal of weight—40 pounds or more. Three of them kept most of the weight off for longer than one year.

Only two of them are still going strong. Their secret? They have learned, on their own, to rid their diets of fat. They also get lots of exercise, walking many miles each day.

We applaud their resolve, but shake our heads knowing that they could have easily and comfortably reached their present situation with the Jack Sprat plan. Like the tortoise, our approach may have taken longer, but it would have been so much more pleasant along the way. We also shake our heads over all the dropouts, many of whom have dashed into other quick weight-loss schemes, including hypnosis.

Is there anything good to say about liquid diets?

Yes. They are good for the economy. The 517 people in the research study spent $1,344,200 on liquid diet programs. Each pound that was lost and kept off for at least one year cost $1,056. Now that's a profit margin!

3

Public Enemy #2

Cigarette smoking is the #1 health problem in America today. The good news is cigarette use is declining in almost all segments of the population. The exception is young females. It's difficult to convince young women who believe "they've come a long way, baby" that they're on a dead-end street.

Unfortunately, consumption of dietary fat—public enemy #2—is not declining at the same rate as cigarette use. This means that in the not too distant future dietary fat will be #1. And when it is, we will find that the war against smoking, difficult as it has been, was a cakewalk compared to the challenge facing us in dietary fat. Smoking can easily be identified as an ugly, stupid, and dangerous habit. Even avid smokers readily admit that smoking gives you dog-breath, stinks up your clothes and hair, yellows your teeth, wrinkles your face, robs your breath, makes you cough, and, of course, kills you.

In contrast, dietary fat is generally viewed as a good guy. Yes, that's right. This cold-blooded mass murderer is viewed as a friend. It has a wonderful public relations team working day and night to promote its image. So successful is this team that every American at his or her core has a powerful bias in favor of dietary fat that is difficult to overcome. Buried in our subconscious minds, thanks to an ingenious PR campaign, is the notion that fat is good.

Who is this dastardly PR team that would promote the positive image of such a heinous substance?

Brace yourself for the answer. It's Mom and Dad!

From the time we are old enough to understand, our parents tell us in every way possible that dietary fat is good stuff. Mom heaps her love on us with generous doses of fat. When we are good, we are rewarded with fat, and when we are bad, fat is withheld. And if mom puts some fat in front of us that we don't want, dad steps in to make certain the deadly stuff is consumed.

That's not true, you say. Only parents who are warped and unfit would do such a thing. Fit parents who really care about their children would protect them with their lives.

True, most parents would fling themselves in front of an oncoming train to save their child's life. Unfortunately, these same parents push health-destroying sludge into their kids at an alarming rate. Worse yet, they try to make the kids believe the sludge is good for them.

Still don't believe us, huh?

Let's look in on a typical American family and we'll show you what we mean. Please feel free to object if you see something that is not a true representation.

It's dinnertime and ten-year-old Johnny sits staring at his plate.

"Come on, Johnny," says Mrs. Smith. "You have to finish your dinner before you get dessert."

Johnny wrinkles his nose.

Mr. Smith speaks up. "Johnny, your mother worked hard making this meal for you, and it's not nice of you to disappoint her by not eating."

Mrs. Smith adds, "And your father worked hard to buy this food for us."

Johnny wrinkles his nose again.

"Okay," Mrs. Smith says soothingly. "You don't have to eat your vegetables and bread, but you do have to eat your meat and drink your milk. Meat and milk will help you grow big and strong."

Mr. Smith adds: "And meat is very expensive. We can't afford to waste it. Money doesn't grow on trees, you know."

Johnny submits to the pressure. He eats his beef, drinks his milk, and is rewarded with chocolate chip cookies for dessert.

Analysis: Johnny's dinner was more than 50 percent fat, and yet he was led to believe that what he ate was good for him. More than that, he was rewarded with fat for eating fat. He also was convinced that vegetables, bread, and the like are inferior foods that are not worth eating.

Our tendencies as parents are formed when we are children. When Johnny grows up, he will likely insist that his children eat their meat and drink their milk. He also will let them slide on the other stuff—the healthy stuff that's low in fat and high in nutrients and fiber.

It's important to point out here that babies and very young children need plenty of dietary fat and cholesterol to help them develop. Well-intentioned parents have created problems by restricting fat intake too early in life. So don't go overboard with your youngsters. At the same time, don't subscribe to the old adage that a fat baby is a healthy baby. In fact, packing on too many pounds early in life can set the stage for obesity later on. Use common sense, and check with your pediatrician before restricting fat intake to a substantial degree. You'll see more on this in mini-chapter 8 in part 3.

It's time for a change, and the cycle must be broken. But don't look for a lot of change any time soon. Too many of us still believe what Mom and Dad taught us when we were growing up. And that's why too many of us are fat and too many of us are at high risk for heart disease, high blood pressure, diabetes, and cancers of the colon, breast, and prostate.

4

Calories Are Not the Problem

Four out of ten American adults currently weigh at least 20 percent more than is thought to be optimal for good health. That comes to roughly 2.5 billion pounds of excess body fat. And things are getting worse, not better. Our frames now carry an additional six pounds of body fat when compared with the 1980 model.

Why has the American waistline been expanding at a rate faster than the national debt? Is it simply a matter of excess calories—eating too much too often?

The answer may surprise you. The average American today does not consume more calories than in 1910. That's not to say there haven't been major changes in the American diet. There have, and the changes have been all bad. Our intake of dietary fat has increased by about 15 percent, and we consume about 20 percent more refined (simple table) sugar. To make matters worse, we have moved toward eating large, infrequent meals as opposed to smaller meals spaced evenly throughout the day.

Surprisingly, millions of Americans are overweight even though their caloric intake is not out of line with their needs. When two groups are placed on 2,000-calorie-a-day diets, the group on the low-fat, high-carbohydrate diet will lose weight.

The high-fat, low-carbohydrate group will not lose weight, and may gain. Obviously, since both groups are consuming the same number of calories, caloric intake cannot be the problem.

Dietary fat makes you fat. It is similar to body fat, and it requires only a tiny biochemical modification before it can be escorted into the storage lockers around your waist, or on your hips, thighs, and buttocks. Only about 3 calories of every 100 calories of fat consumed are required for this modification.

The body treats carbohydrates very differently, and herein lies the crux of the matter. While the body loves to store dietary fat as body fat, it hates to convert carbohydrates to fat, and it will do everything in its power to avoid doing so. Excess calories of carbohydrates are first stored as glycogen—long chains of glucose molecules—in the liver and muscles. But the capacity for storing glycogen is very small, only a few pounds at most, and you quickly reach the limit.

Once you reach the limit, your body will begrudgingly resort to converting carbs to fat. Converting carbs to fat is horribly inefficient, and that's why the body hates doing it. The biochemical processes involved in the conversion exact a heavy price, fully 23 calories out of every 100 calories available. (Remember, the cost for converting fat is only 3 calories per 100.) Multiply this 20-calorie difference times twenty or thirty years, and you see the difference between carbohydrates and dietary fat.

There is another major difference between carbs and fat. Dietary fat comes in concentrated doses of 9 calories per gram, whereas carbohydrates contain only 4 calories per gram. This means you can consume a huge number of calories when you eat even a small amount of fat-laden food. The opposite is true when you eat carbs, and this is one of the basic tenets underlying the Jack Sprat plan.

When we do dietary analyses with our clients, they are often surprised to learn how many calories they are consuming. "But I don't eat that much food," they say. And that's true. But *what* they eat and *when* they eat are making them fat.

Jack Sprat's wife insisted on drinking colas with her meals, while Jack sipped on mineral water with a dash of lime. Jack's wife became obese, and the colas were a big factor. Here's why.

Colas are loaded with refined sugar, which is a sinister accomplice to dietary fat. Refined sugar causes a huge insulin reaction, because it enters the system so quickly. Insulin, in turn, opens the doors of fat cells (connective tissue cells that act as storage lockers for body fat), making them eager to accept fat from the bloodstream.

Combining refined sugar and fat maximizes your ability to store fat. In fact, 5 percent more fat will be stored when sugar and fat are combined, as compared with taking the two separately, even though the number of calories consumed are the same.

Complex sugars, or starch (naturally occurring and found in whole grains, vegetables, and elsewhere), affect the body in a different way. Because they take longer to break down, they filter into the circulation in a "time-released" fashion, leading to a lower concentration of sugar in the blood and a smaller response from the pancreas.

Eating refined sugar and fat together is bad enough, but when you combine the two in large infrequent meals, as many Americans do, you compound the problem. When you eat a lot at one sitting, you cause the pancreas to release a huge dose of insulin. This is true even if what you eat does not contain a large amount of refined sugar. And because the meal was large, there is an abundance of fat to be stored.

What's more, large meals are generally taken at the end of the day, before retiring to the couch or the bedroom. Lack of any sort of physical activity after meals further favors storing incoming fat as body fat.

Looking over this series of events and seeing how typical they are, it's no wonder Americans are fat and getting fatter all the time. It's as if we planned in detail the most efficient ways of storing fat, then set out to maximize those plans. It's time for a change.

5

Low-Fat Limbo

Jack Sprat is a strong supporter of the American Heart Association (AHA). But he doesn't like its stand on dietary fat. He believes that a diet that contains 30 percent fat is not healthy, and he tried to make his case to anyone who would listen. But the U.S. Department of Agriculture and the Surgeon General agreed with the AHA, outnumbering poor Jack. Case closed.

Not quite. The state of knowledge concerning the health consequences of dietary fat supports Jack's position and bolsters the argument for a much lower guideline than the AHA is prepared to back. Ironically, the AHA takes this stand despite advice from its own experts that the guideline should be lower.

A little intrigue here?

Indeed. A few years ago, a panel of distinguished nutritional scientists was charged with formulating dietary guidelines for the AHA. They examined the evidence in great detail, and after careful deliberation, the panel recommended a diet of only 20 percent fat, or less.

But when the recommendation was presented to the powers-that-be, it was rejected. The public won't buy it, the scientists were told. It's too restrictive. And so, the AHA opted for a much higher guideline—not on the basis of the scientific evidence, but on an assumption about what the public would buy into.

In fairness to the powers-that-be, they were probably correct. Recommending that Americans cut their fat intake virtually in half would have been a huge pill to swallow. But at least a legitimate guideline would have been established. As it is, adoption of the 30 percent guideline has caused confusion and harm to the low-fat movement in at least four important ways.

First, whether intended or not, the public views the 30 percent guideline as optimal. This means that if my fat intake is, say, 34 percent, it's only 4 percent away from the optimal level. Hey, no problem! Nobody's perfect. Obviously, 30 percent is much too high to serve as a reference point.

Second, millions of people who desperately need to lower their fat substantially are affected by this guideline. The 30 percent guideline has been adopted not only by the AHA but by the American Diabetes Association and the American Cancer Society.

Third, many scientists use the 30 percent guideline in their research to determine the effects of a "healthy low-fat diet" on breast cancer and other diseases. Not surprisingly, results of such studies have shown little impact. The appropriate conclusion from such studies should be that the AHA guideline is not very effective. Instead, many have concluded, "The data do not support lowering the fat content of the diet as a means to preventing disease."

This is a tremendously important misinterpretation, one that is exploited by medical professionals who oppose preventive health measures in favor of drugs, surgery, and other fix-it approaches. It's like giving a poverty-stricken family a tax cut as an experiment to see if it will improve their standard of living. It won't, of course, and for obvious reason. Even so, if you opposed helping poor people, you could use the results of this experiment to conclude that "helping poor people doesn't change their standard of living, so why bother."

Fourth, the 30 percent guideline has become a smoke screen for special interests. Producers of fatty foods hide behind the fact that you can piece together a diet that is 30 percent fat by counterbalancing their products with low-fat items. You can, for example, eat sausage if you combine it with several pounds of grape skins, giving you an "average" fat content of 30 percent.

Thankfully, there is a strong movement to "redefine" the 30 percent guideline. As a face-saving measure, proponents are now saying that a diet containing 30 percent fat is "transitional." To be healthy, in other words, first drop your fat content to 30 percent, but don't stop there.

The movement toward true low-fat diets is not progressing as quickly as it should. Diehards persist in trying to convince the public that lowering fat consumption is a lot of foolishness, and they jump on every isolated fact and publicize it as proof. Look at the French, they say. They eat as much fat as we do, but their incidence of heart disease is much lower.

The wine industry says the lower incidence is because the French drink a lot of red wine. Fatty food producers say the lower incidence is because dietary fat doesn't count. Neither is correct.

If we trace the fat content of the French diet over the past several decades, we find that it started low and has increased steadily. In 1961, the French consumed about 28 percent of their calories as fat, and it wasn't until 1988 that it reached 39 percent—a level Americans have consumed for more than fifty years. These fifty years are important, because heart disease is a gradual process, building up over decades. The French may be living on borrowed time, and it's possible that an explosion of heart attacks will occur two or three decades from now.

Despite the propaganda of special interests, there is no getting around the wisdom of eating less fat. Medical evidence strongly supports lowering fat intake to no more than 20 percent of total calories. At this level, atherosclerosis (clogging of the arteries) is arrested, and a host of other health-enhancing changes occurs, including the loss of body fat.

Body fat is reduced even when you eat more food. The Chinese are a perfect example. They load up on carbohydrates, mostly complex carbs in the form of rice and vegetables, and they stay slender. In fact, the average Chinese consumes 20 percent more calories than the average American but is 25 percent leaner.

Sounds impossible, doesn't it? But you learned in chapter 2 how this can happen. Eating fat makes you fat; eating carbohydrates keeps you lean. The Chinese eat little red meat—the leading source of dietary fat in the United States—and only 7 percent of their protein comes from animals. Americans consume 33 percent more protein than the Chinese, and 70 percent of our protein comes from animals.

Maybe the Chinese are lean and healthy because they get more exercise than we do. Maybe their lower incidence of heart disease and cancer has nothing to do with fat intake.

Sorry, diehards. True, the Chinese are more physically active than we are. But their leanness and greater health are not owing to excessive exercise. For proof, consider the medical studies of lumberjacks in Finland. These guys get an incredible amount of high-intensity exercise, all day long. And yet, they die at a young age from heart disease. The reason? A diet remarkably high in fat, loaded with cheese and fatty dairy products.

Maybe the Chinese are lean and healthy simply because they are Chinese.

Sorry again. When people from other cultures, including the Chinese, come to this country and become Americanized—eating the way we eat—they get fatter, their health profile plummets, and their risk of heart disease and cancer skyrockets.

If eating a diet that is no more than 20 percent fat is good for your health, are there even more benefits to be accrued from lowering fat intake to 10 percent? The answer is yes. Dean Ornish, M.D., made medical history with his discovery that a 10 percent fat diet combined with other healthful habits (mild exercise, stress management and meditation, group support, and so forth) can reverse atherosclerosis (clogging of the arteries). Nathan Pritikin's plan for healthful living also advocates a 10 percent fat diet. The Pritikin approach claims remarkable transformations among people who follow their plan.

Can you go lower than 10 percent? Yes, but you need to be careful. Your body requires some fat on a daily basis, about 3 percent of total calories. The fat must be in the form of linoleic and linolenic acids—polyunsaturated fats. (See the discussion of various types of fat in chapter 6.)

If you don't get adequate dietary fat, problems can arise. The skin becomes reddened and irritated, infections and dehydration are likely, and liver abnormalities can result. But don't worry. The chances of not getting enough fat in your diet are extraordinarily slim.

In preparing this book, we wondered how Jack Sprat was able to eat *no* fat and still stay so healthy. He told us he didn't know, but he suggested that perhaps a concoction he consumed daily that was passed down for generations among the Sprat men had something to do with it. He gave us the recipe, and we had it analyzed. As it turns out, it contained the exact minimum amount of precisely the kind of fat Jack's body needed.

(When we told Jack the news—that he had, in fact, been eating fat—he became alarmed that some revisionist historian would try to change the nursery rhyme to "Jack Sprat ate a little fat, but mostly he ate lean." We promised him we would keep the secret, and we share it with you confident that you will sustain our promise.)

The Jack Sprat plan is based on an average fat intake of 15 percent. At this level, good things are sure to happen. You may produce faster results with a very-low-fat diet of 10 percent or less, but you also may become discouraged. As a rule of thumb, the greater the change attempted and the further it deviates from what you are accustomed to in your everyday life, the less likely it is to be sustained.

Our advice: adopt the Jack Sprat plan; then kick back and enjoy the flexibility of the diet, the good-tasting foods, and the easier road to success. Take your time, knowing that a year from now, five years from now, a decade from now, you will still be on the plan. Through time, however, you will forget you are on a plan, because it will have become second nature. Good health and a slimmer you will also become second nature. That's our goal, and we believe the odds are in our favor, and yours.

6
All Fats Are Not Created Equal

There are three types of dietary fat: saturated, monounsaturated, and polyunsaturated. All are rich sources of energy, storing 9 calories per gram. Eat too much of any of these three types and you will become fat. But that's where the similarities end.

Saturated fat is a bad dude. It is used by your liver to produce the cholesterol that circulates in your bloodstream. In fact, 80-90 percent of the cholesterol in your blood was produced in your liver with the help of saturated fat. And it's all the bad kind of cholesterol—LDL, the kind that clogs your arteries.

Ironically, eating cholesterol barely raises your serum cholesterol concentration. The body seems to sense that when you increase your intake of cholesterol, it needs to lower production of cholesterol in the liver. The same sort of feedback loop doesn't work with saturated fat, however. The more you take in, the higher your serum cholesterol goes.

This is why a product that is advertised as being "cholesterol-free" won't lower your serum cholesterol, and may in fact raise it if the food contains saturated fat.

Saturated fat is not content merely to promote atherosclerosis. It increases the stickiness of your blood platelets, increasing the likelihood of clot formation. When a clot lodges in a

31

narrowed artery of the heart, you have a heart attack. If the artery is in your brain, you have a stroke. Saturated fat also hikes up your blood pressure and has been linked to diabetes, gallbladder disease, and cancers of the colon, prostate, uterus, and breast.

We cannot overemphasize the evil nature of saturated fat. It is critical that you respect the power of this fiend and its ability to devastate your health, even though you may lower your overall fat intake to a "safe" level. It is imperative that you not only drop your overall fat intake to a maximum of 20 percent but that you also reduce your saturated fat intake as much as possible, the closer to zero the better. The Jack Sprat plan does both for you.

What makes saturated fat so different?

A few hydrogen atoms, that's all. All fats are made up of strings of carbon atoms with hydrogen atoms attached. In saturated fat, all available slots on the carbon chain are filled with hydrogen atoms. The chain is "saturated," in other words. In monounsaturated fat, one available slot on the chain is vacant. In polyunsaturated fat, several of the slots are vacant.

As we told you in the previous chapter, your body requires a modest amount of polyunsaturated fat. It doesn't require the other two types, however, and obviously it would be better off without any saturated fat whatsoever. The problem is we like the taste of foods that contain saturated fat. Think of all the really yummy things you love to eat. Hamburgers, doughnuts, butter, cheese, ice cream, the list goes on. Guess why they are so tasty? You got it. They're loaded with saturated fat.

As if our problems with naturally occurring saturated fat weren't bad enough, we've come up with a way to convert monounsaturated and polyunsaturated fats to saturated fat. The process is called hydrogenation, and it involves adding hydrogen to the vacant slots on the carbon chain that appear in mono and poly fats. Hydrogenation makes a perfectly innocent fat into a criminal, in other words.

Why would we do such a horrible thing?

There are several reasons. When margarine was first introduced, it was liquid at room temperature. Yuk! To please customers, producers hardened margarine by adding hydrogen to polyunsaturated fat. Read margarine labels and you will see items such as "partially hydrogenated soybean oil." This means hydrogen has been added to promote firmness. Peanut butter is smoother and creamier thanks to hydrogenation, and hydrogenated fat takes longer to spoil, thus extending the shelf life.

Hydrogenated fat may be *even more dangerous* than its natural cousin, saturated fat. Recent evidence suggests that the so-called trans fatty acids created in the hydrogenation process do more to increase cholesterol concentration than the saturated fat found naturally in such foods as meat and cheese.

When food is fried in oil, it soaks up fat like a sponge. Americans love fried food, and that's one of the main reasons our intake of fat is so high.

All oils, regardless of type, are all-fat and contain approximately 12 grams of fat and 108 calories per tablespoon. But some oils, especially the "tropical" oils, are high in saturated fat, and should be avoided at all costs.

The principal tropical oils are palm, palm kernel, and coconut oil. Palm oil comes from the fleshy part of the palm plant and contains 6.7 grams of saturated fat per tablespoon. Palm kernel oil comes from the kernel and contains 11.1 grams of saturated fat. Coconut oil is even worse, with 11.8 grams of saturated fat. To give you an idea just how bad these tropical oils are, beef tallow, a well-established villain, contains "only" 6.4 grams of saturated fat per tablespoon.

Coconut oil is everywhere, spreading saturated fat like a plague to places you wouldn't suspect. Years ago, one of our clients, desperate to lower his serum cholesterol level, was advised to do a number of things, including adding oat bran to his diet. Months later, he returned for a blood test to see how he was doing. Despite cutting back on red meat and cheese, his cholesterol was higher than before. He was dumbfounded.

Under questioning, he admitted he didn't like the taste of oatmeal or oat bran, but he had found a great-tasting substitute that he was consuming in large quantities. The substitute was a popular cereal with the words "oat bran" in the name. This cereal contained only a minuscule quantity of oat bran, but the dose of coconut oil was considerable. Ironically, this man had been trying to lower his serum cholesterol by unknowingly consuming huge quantities of saturated fat.

Some of the more conscientious fast-food chains have switched from frying in beef tallow to frying in safflower oil, which is low in saturated fat. The taste is pretty much intact, and the overall fat content is still the same, but the deadly saturated fat content is reduced substantially. Because of consumer concerns, many food manufacturers have decreased the use of tropical oils in cookies and crackers. Unfortunately, many have switched to hydrogenated oils.

Read labels and turn away from products with tropical oils. Sounds simple. It isn't. Many labels state: "Contains one or more of the following: corn oil, soybean oil, palm oil, coconut oil." Obviously, it makes a world of difference if the product is loaded with coconut oil rather than corn oil. But you can't tell from the label which oil is in the product.

Manufacturers claim that more specific labeling would put them at a competitive disadvantage and reduce their profits, because they must be able to respond quickly to market opportunities. When corn is plentiful and cheap, corn oil is used in the product. When coconuts are cheaper, coconut oil is used. Changing from one oil to another occurs quickly, and there isn't time to change labels. Or so manufacturers say. And unfortunately, despite new laws governing labeling, don't look for this to change.

7

Sleuth, Then Slash

In Jack Sprat's heyday, everyone believed that starches made you fat and that meat and dairy products were healthy and kept you lean. In fact, Little Miss Muffet's restaurant used to serve a diet plate that contained a large ground-beef patty plus a mound of rich cottage cheese. Bread and potatoes were forbidden, of course.

These beliefs fed the mystery of why Jack stayed so lean while his wives became immense, because Jack ate at least a loaf of bread each day, plus stacks of potatoes.

Miss Muffet's so-called diet plate was a horrible blend of fatty foods that, if anything, would help you gain weight. But it looked so healthy and lean. That's the problem with dietary fat. It's not limited to the edges of choice prime rib. It's all over the place, and it turns up in the most unexpected places.

In our workshops, when we start talking about dietary fat and all the problems it causes, we can tell by the looks on people's faces that they're thinking: "Not me—I don't eat much fat." But when we tell them where the fat comes from, their looks change. They know they have been eating a whole lot more fat than they thought.

So where is all this fat?

Here are the top sources of fat in the American diet. But before we list them, keep a few reference points in mind. First, the average American diet is 35-40 percent fat. That's 90-120 grams of fat per day, or 20-27 teaspoons. A healthy body-fat-reducing diet should contain less than half that amount of fat, or less than 40 grams *per day*. Use this as a reference point when you review the top five sources of fat below.

1. **Ground beef products**
    (hamburgers, cheeseburgers, and meatloaf)
    *   small hamburger = 9 grams of fat
        (add cheese = 13 grams of fat)
    *   double giant burger with cheese = 61 grams of fat
2. **Processed meats, including luncheon meats and hot dogs**
    *   3.5 ounce serving of salami = 21 grams of fat
    *   3.5 ounce serving of sausage = 27 grams of fat
    *   3.5 ounce serving of bologna = 30 grams of fat
    *   hot dog (about 1 ounce of meat) = 10-17 grams of fat
    *   giant hot dog = as high as 25 grams of fat
3. **Whole milk and whole milk products**
    *   one cup (half-pint carton) of whole milk = 8 grams of fat
    *   one cup of 2 percent milk = 5 grams of fat
    *   milk shakes = 15-20 grams of fat
    *   one ounce of cheese = about 9 grams of fat
4. **Doughnuts, cookies and cakes**
    (baked goods often are deep fried or loaded with butter and oils)
    *   one glazed doughnut = 10 to 25 grams of fat
    *   one croissant = 19 grams of fat
5. **Beef steaks and roasts**
    *   3.5 ounce serving of "lean" pot roast = 10 grams of fat
    *   3.5 ounce serving of ribeye steak = 12 grams of fat
    *   3.5 ounce serving of short ribs = 18 grams of fat
        Note: a 3.5-ounce serving is extremely small (less than a typical lunch serving).

Don't think that fat oozes only from these five leading sources. All fried foods are packed with fat. Take commercially prepared fried chicken, for example. A center breast piece contains 15 grams of fat. If we order this piece extra crispy, the fat content jumps to 20 grams. Remember, that's just *one* breast. French fries also are loaded with fat. A small order of fast-food fries contains 12 grams of fat, a medium order contains 17 grams, and a large contains 22 grams.

Many restaurants make a big deal out of changing their frying habits from beef tallow to safflower or corn oil. This is an important move because it reduces the saturated fat content of fried foods. But remember, all fat, regardless of the type, contains 9 calories per gram. All fat makes you fat, in other words. And when you get fat, you increase your risks of high blood pressure, heart disease, and diabetes.

Chocolate is another major source of fat, as are salad oils, mayonnaise, peanut butter, and many other foods. The point is, fat is everywhere, and you must be vigilant in your quest to lower the fat content of your diet. Fortunately, the Jack Sprat plan will do that for you.

Counting fat grams is one way of monitoring your fat intake. The Jack Sprat plan will keep your fat grams under control. Another useful way of looking at food is by determining what percentage of fat it contains. Knowing percentages will help you make quick judgments about whether a food ought to be included in your diet.

Food producers provide everything you need to know about their products, except the percentage of fat per serving. But you can figure that for yourself. It's easy.

Let's turn that half-pint carton of whole milk over and see what the label tells us. First, we find that there are 8 grams of fat per serving and 150 calories. There's one other piece of information you need to know, but it's not on the label. Fat contains 9 calories per gram. Remember that! Now, here are the simple calculations:

8 grams of fat contain 72 calories
(8 grams x 9 cals/gram = 72 calories)

This means that of the total of 150 calories, 72 are from fat. To find the percentage:

Divide 72 by 150 = .48, or 48 percent.

Whole milk is 48 percent fat. Wouldn't it be helpful if the label told us that?

Next time you're at the market, look at the label on "2% low-fat" milk and do some calculations. You will find that it is 37.5 percent fat. That's hardly low in fat, and that's why consumer protection groups have for years been battling the dairy industry to remove the "low-fat" label from 2 percent milk.

When you see a food label that says "97% fat-free," you are likely to think that the product is healthy because it is very low in fat. Be careful. You may be stepping into a trap. The reason is, many food manufacturers report the fat content of their products by weight, not by calories, and the implications are tremendous.

When fat is reported by weight, it is totally meaningless to the consumer. Why do it then? Because it allows a product that is loaded with fat to appear much leaner than it actually is. The perfect example is milk.

Whole milk by weight is only 3.3 percent fat, but 48 percent fat by calories. The difference is caused by the high water content of milk, a fact that producers use to their advantage. Water has no calories or nutrients, and nutritionists remove water when making their decisions about fat content. According to milk producers, whole milk qualifies for a "96.7% fat-free" label. According to nutritionists, it qualifies for only a "52% fat-free" label. Doesn't sound nearly as good, does it? Smart money says listen to the nutritionists.

The same ruse is used by meat producers, because meat has a high water content. Sludge-laden sausage that is more than 80 percent fat may have a label that reads, "76% fat-free," for example.

How can you protect yourself?

Do some quick math, taking into consideration the fat grams and total calories per serving as described above. When you do, you will immediately see the trickery. But meats and several other products often don't have traditional labels, and they don't tell you the fat content in grams or the total calories per serving. When there are no labels, or when the information is incomplete, the only way you can protect yourself is by being suspicious.

Flimflammers depend on our trusting nature. Disregard all percent fat-free claims as bogus, unless there is information on the label to back it up. If sufficient information is not available, assume the worst, move on, and buy something else you're sure of.

New laws will give us new labels. Are the new labels a big improvement? Unfortunately, no. They are not nearly as useful as they could be. Percentages are included, but they do not represent the percentage of fat contained in the food. For example, a food label on a box of macaroni and cheese shows 13 grams of fat per serving, and adjacent to the 13 grams on the label is a percentage (20%).

What does this percentage mean?

Is the product 20 percent fat? No. Actually, it is 46 percent fat. The 20 percent fat is the proportion of the total daily recommended fat intake. This means the 13 grams of fat represents 20 percent of the total daily fat intake of 65 grams.

Is this confusing?

Of course it is. Not only that, these computations are based on a diet that is 30 percent fat. You learned in chapter 3 that 30 percent fat is not a low-fat diet. Certainly, consuming 65 grams of fat per day does not pave the way to reduced body fat and health. But that's the way it is. Again, we say, buyer beware. (For more information on the new labeling system, see mini-chapter 19.)

8

80-20 and the Warthogs

Does going on the Jack Sprat plan mean you will never again experience the joys of cheesecake or fried chicken? Will holidays be a drag, watching others stuff themselves to their heart's content with holiday goodies while you pick away at the celery and carrot sticks?

Admittedly, holidays can be tough, and for that reason we recommend that you not try to start on the Jack Sprat plan during the Thanksgiving to New Year's holiday season. The cravings and fond memories of sludge-filled family get-togethers will defeat you before you get out of the starting block. Wait until January 2. And by the time next year's holiday season rolls around, you will be ready to cope with it.

That's not to say that on the Jack Sprat plan you will forever be lurking about salad bars picking at raw broccoli. You will, in fact, be eating more food than ever before. That's important to know, because when you are hungry you crave old favorites—the kinds of food Mom gave you when you were a kid that made you feel all warm and cozy.

The Jack Sprat plan is loaded with foods that will fool you. They look fatty, and they taste good. They should satisfy most of your cravings; however, we are not so naive that we believe all cravings will go away. They won't. But we have that covered.

The plan allows an occasional indulgence. We call it "controlled cheating." This aspect differs greatly from other programs, which insist on strict compliance. The problem with such a rigid approach is that once the dam breaks, guilt overtakes you and there's no going back.

During your early days on the Jack Sprat plan, before you have fully embraced new habits and a new perspective, you will be tempted by old favorites. That's natural. And the more you are tempted and the more you refuse, the greater the temptation will become. That's why we say give in to it. Declare a "warthog" day and go for it.

Your progress should not be slowed appreciably because of warthog days, if you don't overdo it. To lessen the negative effects, we have prepared guidelines for you. On the Jack Sprat plan you will have four warthog days from which to choose such items as pizza, fried chicken, Mexican food, and a big burger and fries. Each warthog day adds 500 calories above your assigned rate, plus additional fat grams. But the fat content of a warthog day does not exceed 30 percent, and often is much lower.

Warthogging in this fashion—with a relatively low fat intake—will do the least damage while satisfying your needs.

Use warthog days only when you have to. Do not schedule them, because you run the risk of sitting around fantasizing about burritos and burgers. We recommend that you wait until you feel yourself in the grasp of a Big Mac attack, then succumb. Knowing you can give in to the urge is often enough to allay it.

Please don't assume that we are encouraging you to use warthog days. On the contrary, we firmly believe you can get by quite well without them. But like a life jacket, they are there for emergencies, and they will help keep you moving in the right direction.

In order to minimize negative effects, it is important that you limit your warthogging to warthog days only, rather than extending your indulgence over several days. Your body can cope more effectively with one major pig-out than it can with a series of smaller transgressions. This is true even though total caloric and fat gram intakes are the same. You are better off eating the entire 10-ounce bag of peanut M&M's in one sitting, in other words, than to pick at them 1 or 2 ounces at a time over several days.

When you have arrived at the point where you are pretty satisfied with your weight and your health profile, you can fall off the wagon more often without ill effects. We call this the 80-20 rule. If 80 percent of the time you are eating the right things, ill-advised indulgences 20 percent of the time won't be a major problem. That 20 percent of the time, by the way, will get you very nicely through next year's holiday season. But for the novice who is striving to reach a goal, you'd better stick to the 95-5 rule, which allows only an occasional warthog day.

An interesting thing happens to your taste buds when you follow a low-fat diet for a prolonged period of time. They become keener. On your old high-fat diet, your taste buds were dulled by a constant flow of rich-tasting sludge. As with addictive drugs, you had to increase the sludge quotient in order to get your kicks. That's why desserts such as double-fudge brownies with ice cream topped with melted chocolate and whipped cream are so popular.

But after eating the Jack Sprat way, you will find that your taste buds are more easily satisfied. This effect cuts two ways. Your taste buds will, on the one hand, demand less fat in foods. When, on the other hand, they encounter a rich, sludge-filled delight, the taste will seem almost cosmic.

Won't this inspire you to pursue more fatty delights?

Surprisingly, no. Changes in your perspective on eating plus changes in your gastrointestinal tract won't allow it. In the old days, you could eat sludge for days on end without feeling the effects because you probably never felt all that good anyway—at least not as good as you could have. But on the Jack Sprat plan, you will be used to feeling good, and when you don't, you won't like it. You won't like the way sludge makes you sluggish, causes you to feel overstuffed, and seems to stay forever in your gut. You especially won't like the effects you will feel after eating something greasy.

Eventually, Jack Sprat will win you over completely, and you will marvel at the way you used to eat.

9
Smart Choices

Jack Sprat never needed to diet, and despite his voracious appetite and ability to outeat everyone in the county, he stayed slim and trim. He didn't have to diet because the food he ate was so low in fat, and he loved it. Good for him. But what about the rest of us, scourged from birth with taste buds that crave fat every waking hour? Is there any hope?

Of course there is, and that's the beauty of the Jack Sprat plan. Just give it a shot for 28 days, and you will be hooked.

To get you off on the right foot, you have to become knowledgeable about the issues and what's at stake. You will get that from reading the chapters in this book and from the experience you will gain during your 28 days on the plan. After that, you will be armed with everything you need to make smart choices.

So what's a smart choice? Wiring your jaws shut? Switching to an all-liquid diet? Cutting daily calories to fewer than 1,000?

Not even close. A smart choice is one that pays dividends without demanding sacrifices (of health, well-being, or comfort). The dividends may be small, but taken collectively over time, dividends add up and make a substantial difference. Here is an example of the advantage of a common everyday smart choice over a not-so-smart choice.

Not-so-smart choice. A small vending-machine size Snickers candy bar (2.07 oz.) contains 280 calories and 14 grams of fat. Yum-yum! Rip open the wrapper and wolf down the contents. Average taste bud titillation time? For men, three bites, 12.6 seconds. Women, on the other hand, tend to extend their pleasure, nibbling at the chocolate concoction. The duration is longer, but the intensity factor is reduced greatly.

Smart choice. A McDonald's low-fat hot fudge sundae contains nearly the same number of calories (290), but has only 5 grams of fat. Yum-yum! No sacrifice here. But there are dividends: (1) the taste bud titillation time is longer than the vending machine alternative, and the intensity is just as great; (2) the sundae is not as destructive to health, because the fat content is nearly three times lower; (3) over one year, saving only 9 grams of fat per day (without cutting calories) could add up to more than a pound of fat lost from the body.

The McDonald's sundae demonstrates that fast-food items can be included in a low-fat eating plan. But be careful of look-alikes. Other fast-food hot fudge sundaes may contain more than 300 calories and 10 or more grams of fat (half of which are saturated fat). Clearly, they are not-so-smart choices.

It is imperative that you be able to distinguish between smart choices and not-so-smart choices. Too often, the dividing line is blurry, and false claims and advertisements make it even more blurry. This book will be your bifocals, helping you to see clearly and focus on where you want to be, and it will help you get there comfortably.

Fortunately, it's getting easier to go low-fat, and much of the battle can be won by making better choices. But how will you know what choices to make? At this point, you already have a pretty good idea. But to help you move farther along, we provide a wide range of smart choices in Resource 4. Switching from tuna salad made with mayonnaise, for example, to tuna salad made with Kraft Free mayonnaise or fat-free plain yogurt dressing will save you a whopping 11 grams of fat per serving. That could be (depending on your weight and level of physical activity) 25 percent or more of a full day's allotment of dietary fat.

Many people who see the Jack Sprat plan for the first time

are amazed at the amount of food it allows you to eat each day. They say, "I never eat that much! If I did, I'd be big as a blimp!" It's true. They would be big as a blimp if they ate that much of the kinds of food they are used to eating. Making smart choices allows you to eat more.

Surely, you might say, the Jack Sprat plan is more difficult than it looks.

Not so. Rob, an executive from Louisville, was resistant to the Jack Sprat message. He subscribed to the eat, drink, and be merry philosophy, and he wasn't about to sacrifice his "quality" of life in the interests of enhanced health. Giving up cheeseburgers was not even open for discussion. But during a workshop we convinced him that if he wanted to continue making merry, he'd better give some thought to his health-destroying habits. When we saw him weeks after the workshop, he called from a distance: "It ain't that hard!" Then he walked up, smiled, and said: "This low-fat business is just not that difficult." Rob was eating more—"grazing," we call it—and enjoying his eating. He had lost a dozen pounds, his cholesterol had dropped substantially, and he was feeling better than he had in years. He was simply making smarter choices.

10
Eat, Drink, and Be Active

In our workshops, we have found that people are eager for information about heart disease, stress, body fat, dietary fat, and how to eat smart. But when we mention the word *exercise,* eyes glaze over and a hushed silence fills the room. You can read their minds. "Here comes another pep talk on the benefits of jogging. Rah! Rah! Rah! Listen to Nike and 'Just Do It!' "

The fitness movement has been around for twenty-five years, and most of us at one time or another have tried jogging, cycling, rowing, swimming laps, or cross-country skiing. And after trying it, 92 percent of us said, "No thanks." We found that it was too boring, too exhausting, too time-consuming, too painful. And because we said, "No thanks," most of us carry a twinge of guilt that pecks at us, reminding us that we should be out there, huffing, puffing, and sweating, and that when we are not, we are shirking our duty. No wonder we turn a deaf ear to anyone who wants to talk about exercise.

Fortunately, there is a new message to ease our guilt and get us moving again. But before sharing this message, we must emphasize that medical research is uncompromising about exercise. You must be physically active! No ifs, ands, or buts about it.

Now the good news. It is the *process* of being physically active that counts when it comes to being healthy, looking good, and feeling good. The *product*—physical fitness—is less important. Concentrating on the process instead of the product opens up a whole smorgasbord of opportunities.

Exercise can take the form of everyday activities such as walking, gardening, golf, and other light sporting activities, or washing the car, cutting the grass, and other household chores. All physical activity counts.

This is a very different message from the one aerobic advocates have given us. For twenty-five years we have been told to drive our heart rate up to a target zone and keep it there for at least twenty minutes. If we didn't do this, our exercise wasn't doing us any good. A six-block errand to the grocery store was a waste of time unless we jogged to the store, jogged up and down the aisles, jogged in place during checkout, then jogged home. And if we got home too soon, we had to jog in place on the porch, knowing that if we stopped one second shy of twenty minutes we received absolutely no benefit whatsoever.

And when it came to cutting the grass or washing the car we opted to hire the kid next door, because everyone knew you couldn't keep your heart rate up in the target zone the whole time you were washing or mowing. Ironically, this fitness dogma has been one of the strongest contributors to the current bumper crop of American couch potatoes.

Medical science now confirms that moderate, comfortable, convenient physical activity can improve your health and help you lose weight. Taking a walk or playing badminton does you as much good as jogging. The difference is, walking and badminton won't increase your fitness the way jogging will. But for the 92 percent of us who don't enjoy jogging, rowing, or swimming laps—walking and badminton don't require that you huff and puff and sweat bullets either.

All physical activity burns calories. A comfortable 2-mile walk in the woods burns as many calories as a 1.5-mile exhausting run. When it comes to weight management and health, it's the number of calories you burn that counts. With this in mind, it makes a lot of sense to enjoy your physical activity along the way, by choosing things that are easy and convenient and that you like to do.

Exercise on the job counts too. UPS delivery workers burn an extraordinary number of calories during the course of an eight-hour shift, stepping up and down from the truck, climbing stairs, walking in bursts. So why aren't all UPS workers lean? Unfortunately, like Jack Sprat's wives, they eat the fat, and short of training for a marathon, no amount of daily exercise can cancel out a diet loaded with fat.

When physically active people, like UPS workers, switch to the Jack Sprat plan, they change dramatically in a very short period of time. The combination of a low-fat diet plus huge doses of physical activity works wonders.

But you don't have to get megadoses of exercise to lose body fat and improve your health profile on the Jack Sprat plan. All you have to do is get your body moving on a regular basis. In the next chapter, we will tell you how to move smartly in order to maximize the effects of exercise with a minimum of time and effort.

In the meantime, we need to take stock of where you are right now in your physical activity habits. It's an important consideration because it determines the number of calories your body requires each day to sustain your present weight. We will use this information in part 2, but we want to get you thinking about it now. Place yourself in one of the following four categories. Be honest. And be conservative in your assessment: if you err, err toward the down side (the less active side). The vast majority of Americans will fall within the first two categories.

Couch potato: You specialize in avoiding physical activity, and you limit yourself to things like walking short distances to and from your car—to the office or the house—and once inside, your movement is limited. Evenings and weekends are more likely to find you in front of the TV than outside.

Mild activity: You don't go out of your way to add exercise to your life, but you don't avoid it either. You are somewhat active on the job and/or around the house. This means you spend at least a portion of the work day on your feet—frequently (several times per hour) running errands on the job or engaging in typical household chores at home. Weekends find you outside at least part of the time, in the garden, walking in the park, washing the car, cutting the grass, engaging in light sporting activities such as golf, and so forth.

Moderate activity: In addition to the items associated with "mild activity," you incorporate exercise into your daily routine in the amount of approximately one hour per day. The exercise is brisk but not terribly demanding—brisk walking or light jogging, aerobics classes, moderate sporting activities such as basketball, squash, or tennis. On weekends you are likely to be very physically active. A highly active job, such as being a waitress, carpenter, or delivery person, in which you are on your feet and moving will get you into this category.

Heavy activity: If you engage in heavy aerobic training (running an hour or more per day) or if you are employed in heavy industry (construction, foundry work, and such), you will require a substantial number of calories to sustain your weight. But this category should be reserved only for those who perform intensive and prolonged exercise on a daily basis.

Now that you have selected a category, jot it down and keep it handy. You will need to refer to your category in chapter 12.

II

Beyond Afterburn

Jack Sprat and his wife ate their meals together and labored together in the fields. They were inseparable with only one exception, and that exception turned out to be important. It is the basis for the Jack Sprat Smart Exercise plan.

Every day, after lunch and dinner, Jack would go for a walk. Not a long walk or a fast walk. Just a comfortable walk over the hills and dales, during which he enjoyed the scenery and chatted with passersby. Mrs. Sprat, on the other hand, always retired immediately for a nap. She was woozy, you see, from eating all that fat, and she simply had to lie down for a while. It's a shame Jack never knew that his wife's napping helped make her fat.

When you eat fat, it goes from your stomach into your digestive tract, and from there into your bloodstream. As it circulates in your blood, you have the perfect opportunity to use it as fuel. If you don't, it finds its way into fat cells and is stored, and once stored it is difficult to dislodge. Napping after meals maximizes storage.

Exercise after meals minimizes fat storage, but postmeal exercise has been discouraged during the fitness craze of the past two decades. And for good reason. *Vigorous* exercise after meals is a no-no because working muscles compete with the digestive tract for blood flow, and the muscles always win. (In early times, outrunning a vicious beast was considered more important than adequately digesting your last meal.) When blood goes to the muscles, it is rerouted away from the gut, resulting in discomfort and possibly painful cramping. You no doubt remember Mom telling you not to go swimming after eating because you would get cramps and drown. It's true. In fact, during heavy exercise, especially exercise involving lifting, an extended stomach caused by a large meal can make breathing more difficult and may even interfere with heart function.

The aerobics movement has insisted that we always exercise on an empty stomach, at least two and preferably three hours after eating. When you exercise on an empty stomach, you have to pry open fat cells, drag fat out of storage and into the bloodstream, then deliver it to the muscles where it is used as fuel. This is not an efficient approach to using fat as fuel, and it may reduce the amount of fat you use in favor of more easily available carbohydrate.

This means that mild exercise is not only as good as heavy exercise but in some cases may be even better. You can perform mild exercise after meals, using fat (as fuel) that is pouring into the bloodstream from the meal you just consumed. Smart money says burn off as much of this fat as you can, because the more you use as fuel, the less will be available for storage. We call this "vacuuming" the blood.

There is more to the story. First, don't think you have to get up from the table and immediately start exercising. As long as you exercise within about an hour after eating, you will still get the benefits. Second, because you can perform only mild exercise after eating, this ensures that you will optimize the fuel mix in favor of fat.

The beauty of postmeal exercise is that it is similar to having eaten less fat. Even a small bout of exercise after eating acts to reduce the impact of the fat you have just eaten. In this way, on the Jack Sprat plan you can, in effect, lower the fat content of the diet even further, achieving the benefits of a very-low-fat intake, without restricting yourself at the lunch and dinner table to the extent that would normally be required.

Here is an example of how you can lower the Jack Sprat 15 percent fat diet to 10 percent without eating less fat. On the plan, if you were consuming 2,000 calories per day, you would be consuming 34 grams of fat. If you took a brisk walk at 3.0 mph for 20 minutes after both lunch and dinner (covering a total of two miles), you would expend approximately 200 calories. At least half of those calories, or 100, would come from fat, the remaining 100 would come from carbohydrate. The 100 calories from fat represent slightly more than 11 grams of fat (remember: fat contains 9 calories per gram). If we subtract the 11 grams of fat from the daily allotment of 34, we end up with 23. Your body has to contend with only 23 grams of fat, in other words, and not 34. This would reduce the percentage of fat in the diet from 15 percent to 10 percent. That's a tremendous change, and it's all because you walked a comfortable mile after lunch and after dinner.

But that's not all of the advantages to postmeal mild exercise. In addition:

- It aids digestion, helping move foodstuffs through the bowels.
- It perks you up. You feel exhilarated instead of "draggy," and it has a special calming effect on your mind.
- It adds a 10 percent bonus to the cost of exercise. Walking a mile would normally burn 100 calories, but, after a meal, the walk would burn 110 calories.
- It adds an additional 5 percent bonus by maintaining the metabolic rate at a higher level when the exercise is finished. This is called the afterburn, and we now know that the afterburn burns hotter when exercise is performed on a full stomach. This ups the cost of that one-mile walk from 100 to 115 calories.
- It can prevent a serious health danger called the "Last Supper Syndrome."

What is the "Last Supper Syndrome"? When fat enters the circulation after a meal it activates Factor VII, which triggers the release of blood-clotting substances. The greater the amount of fat entering the circulation, the greater the release of Factor VII and the greater the likelihood that clots will form in the bloodstream. This is a potentially lethal situation, because small blood clots can lodge in areas of an artery that have been narrowed because of atherosclerosis. If a clot lodges in an artery feeding the heart, it stops the flow of blood. Blood carries oxygen, and without oxygen the heart muscle will die. This is called a myocardial infarction, or heart attack. If the same thing happens in the brain, it is called a stroke.

On the Jack Sprat plan it is recommended that you invest at least 10-15 minutes exercising after lunch and dinner. Make a commitment to do this faithfully, and it will pay big dividends. We emphasize exercise after lunch and dinner because after breakfast it's rush, rush, rush, and there is no time for anything, especially a bout of blood-vacuuming, health-promoting exercise. For that reason, breakfasts on the Jack Sprat plan are essentially fat-free. The major fat intake, such as it is, will come from lunch and dinner.

The amount of after-meal exercise we are recommending should fit comfortably into the lunch hour. And we recommend that the last meal of the day be taken relatively early in the evening to allow plenty of time for exercise before you settle in. A low-fat snack taken later will kill any hunger pangs that may arise. We realize that at times it will be difficult to follow through, but if you are in a pinch, any little bit of exercise—a few flights of stairs at a slow pace or a walk around the block—helps.

For those of you who are likely to succumb to guilt when you can't exercise, here is a point to keep in mind. The Jack Sprat plan will work whether or not you include Smart Exercise. So don't despair if you have trouble being perfect. Simply know that exercise optimizes what Jack Sprat has to offer. It will help you get to where you want to go faster. But without it, you will get there anyway; it'll just take a little longer.

Choose exercise that is comfortable and convenient. Walking is probably the best choice, but feel free to use your imagination. The key is to move your body and keep it moving. Because the intensity of what you choose to do will be low, you don't have to change your clothes or your shoes, and you don't have to shower afterwards. This keeps the time commitment to a minimum.

Here are some guidelines that will help you plan your Smart Exercise program. We make the assumption that the intensity of your exercise is approximately that of a 3.5 mph walk. This is the speed of a moderately brisk walk—the speed you would use when changing planes in an airport, assuming that you are not pinched for time. Compare other activities you might choose with this reference. You should not choose any type of exercise that is more demanding. For exercise that is less demanding, lower your allotment of calories and fat grams by your best estimate (10 percent, 20 percent, etc.).

You will note that the Smart Exercise Table is not gender-based. The number of calories and the number of fat grams you burn per minute are driven by body weight.

1. Find your present weight in the Smart Exercise Table.

2. Determine the number of total calories and the amount of fat (in grams) you would burn per minute during postmeal exercise. Numbers in the table include bonus calories accorded postmeal exercise.

3. Multiply this number by the number of minutes you exercise to determine the total number of calories and fat grams expended.

4. Example: A 130-pound person would expend 5.3 calories per minute of exercise. Since the exercise is mild, the fuel mix favors fat to the greatest extent possible. This means that 50 percent of the total calories are derived from the burning of fat: that's 2.6 calories from fat per minute. This equates to .29 grams of fat per minute.

If a 15-minute walk were taken after lunch, and another 15-minute walk were taken after dinner, the 30 minutes of total exercise would expend:

30 x 5.3 calories = 159 calories; and
30 x .29 grams = 8.7 grams of fat.

5. There are two ways you can look at the fat you burn on the Smart Exercise plan. One, you can view it as helping you reach your goal sooner. Or two, you can use these fat grams as a piggy bank, saving them up for a warthog day (more on this in

Smart Exercise Table

PRESENT WEIGHT	TOTAL CALORIES PER MINUTE	FAT CALORIES PER MINUTE	FAT GRAMS PER MINUTE
100-120	4.7	2.4	.27
121-140	5.3	2.6	.29
141-160	5.6	2.8	.31
161-180	6.1	3.1	.34
181-200	6.8	3.4	.37
201-220	7.1	3.5	.39
221+	7.4	3.7	.41

part 2). This might make the journey a little longer, but it will make it a little more pleasant along the way.

What if you exercised for two hours or more after meals, burning off a lot of calories and a lot of fat? Could you get to the point where you were burning off too much incoming fat and not leaving enough for your body's needs?

The answer is no. You would not be able to capture all the fat you had just consumed. Picture hundreds of baby chicks that are released into a field. They run off in all directions, and you try your best to catch them before they reach the tall grass. But try as you will, you can't possibly catch them all. The same is true for the fat you have just eaten. Enough will escape from your exercising muscles to meet your needs in the skin and elsewhere. As we told you in chapter 3, not getting enough fat in their diet is about as likely for Americans as getting hit by a red, white, and blue meteorite on the Fourth of July.

A word of caution: Beware of enthusiasm. When you see how well things are progressing, you may be tempted to work harder and do more. This must be avoided. When you push yourself, you lower the use of fat as fuel, and that is counterproductive when exercising after a meal.

You also risk burnout. Remember, you are trying to establish new lifestyle patterns, and the easier the new patterns are for you, the more likely they are to be sustained. After your postlunch or postdinner exercise, you should be thinking: "Is that all there is to it? Gee, that wasn't much at all."

The aerobic fitness movement taught us that exercise was painful work. That's why it failed most of us. Now we know better. You don't have to huff and puff and sweat bullets to get plenty of benefits from exercise. On the contrary, the easy route is the smart route.

Part Two
The Diet Plan

12

Target Weight

To plug into the Jack Sprat plan, you first must determine the number of daily calories your body requires. Your number will be personalized as much as possible (without an excess of scientific manipulation and calculation) in terms of gender, size, age, physical activities, and goals. This approach differs from most other diets, which put everyone on the same plan and simply slash caloric intake to starvation levels. The starvation approach ensures rapid weight loss. But that's precisely what you don't want to happen because, as you are now aware, weight that is lost in a hurry is mostly muscle and water.

Selecting an appropriate number of daily calories is critical, and it requires delicate balancing. You must, on the one hand, consume a sufficient amount of energy to sustain muscle mass and water balance. This is important because when you lose muscle, your metabolic rate plummets, and body fat loss is stymied (see mini-chapters on "Body Fat"). But, on the other hand, you don't want to consume too many calories because excess calories also will interfere with fat loss. Finding the balancing point is the key, and that is our intention.

Selecting an accurate daily caloric intake for you also is critical because it determines the number of fat grams you will consume each day. This, of course, is the heart of the Jack Sprat plan.

The Jack Sprat plan uses an innovative approach. Your daily caloric intake will be commensurate with the metabolic needs required to sustain your target weight, *not* your present weight. Your target weight is your present weight minus the number of pounds of fat you wish to lose.

Determining your target weight is very easy. It's simply the weight you want to be. But you must be reasonable when making this decision. A good reference point is your weight when you were a young adult (approximately twenty-one years of age) plus 3 percent for each decade beyond your twenties, up to a total of 9 percent. Thus, you would add 3 percent to the weight you were as a young adult if you are in your thirties, 6 percent if you are in your forties, and so forth. This assumes, of course, that you were satisfied with your weight as a young adult.

When you calculate your target weight, you may find that it isn't low enough to suit you. Some clients have told us that when they added 9 percent to their weight as a young adult, the result was a weight that was too close to their present weight—a weight that was not satisfactory to them. In that case, simply knock off a few more pounds to suit yourself. Remember, the target weight is the weight you want to be. We are only trying to help you make the decision in an informed way and reach a realistic and attainable number.

If you were not satisfied with your weight as a young adult, obviously you don't want to use that weight as a target. Instead, simply subtract a reasonable number of pounds from your present weight. If your weight has been a problem for many years, you probably have a good idea of how many pounds need to come off.

Please note: as we have mentioned before, we don't want you to become weight-conscious. The purpose of choosing a target weight is to have a meaningful reference point from which to make decisions regarding the appropriate number of calories and fat grams for you. Once this is established, get rid of the scale and don't think about how many pounds you are losing. When you are settled into the Jack Sprat diet, everything will take care of itself.

Whether you use your weight as a young adult as a reference or not, your target weight should not be more than 40 pounds lower than your present weight. If you are more than 40 pounds overweight, it will be necessary for you to progress in stages. Your first target will be 40 pounds less than you are now. When you reach that target, it will be time to set a new target and begin the process again with a new and lower caloric and fat gram intake.

On the Jack Sprat plan, you will develop eating habits that will sustain your target weight. Eating to sustain your target weight will ensure that you are consuming lots of complex carbohydrates and sufficient protein, providing energy to keep your muscles happy and to preserve water balance. But, because your target weight is lower than your present weight, your body will need to tap into its stored fat in order to meet overall energy demands. This is especially evident on the Jack Sprat plan, because your dietary fat intake will be quite low and you will increase your physical activity after meals.

Eating to sustain your *target* weight is an important innovation, because it means the Jack Sprat plan is both a *weight loss* and a *weight maintenance* plan. After reaching your goal, there is no need to switch to a maintenance diet, which means you won't be abandoning the good habits you developed on the plan. This is important, because the more often you change, the less likely you are to succeed in the long run.

What if you change your mind and no longer want to dedicate yourself to reaching your target weight?

We doubt that this will happen, because we have placed a lid of 40 pounds on your goal setting. Even so, we are aware that lofty goals can inspire initially, then discourage. If you decide along the way that your target weight is too far out of reach and the road too demanding, change your goal. Adjust your target weight upward and increase your caloric intake and fat grams accordingly. Don't be afraid to experiment with various targets in order to determine which will work for you.

Whatever you do, don't accuse yourself of failure. On the contrary, despite our attempts to help you avoid unreasonable expectations, your original goal may have been too far away. Or you may have discovered that you are perfectly satisfied at a weight that exceeds your target. Congratulations! Precious few of us are satisfied with our weight. And you will be healthier because you're not consuming as much fat.

As you proceed, the sophistication of the Jack Sprat plan may seem somewhat complex and too scientific. But actually, it's quite simple. Take your time while we walk you through it. Have a pencil ready to jot things down as you go along. A calculator may come in handy too.

Keep in mind that you are learning new habits and discovering new tools you will use for the rest of your life. Once you learn them and use them, they are yours forever. That's why we want to make certain you get off on the right foot.

The first step is to be as accurate as possible in setting your daily caloric intake. This doesn't mean that you have to be unduly meticulous in your daily eating so that you consume an exact number of calories. That would be impossible. There is no system short of confining you to a metabolic ward in the hospital that can assure precise caloric intake. But a reasonable amount of accuracy, which can be achieved quite easily, is necessary for success.

Our primary reason for insisting upon accuracy in setting daily caloric intake is that this information will determine the number of fat grams you should consume in order to reach your goal. Fat gram intake is the backbone of the Jack Sprat plan, and you need to commit yourself to consuming only your assigned number of fat grams per day. The better you are at doing this, the more successful you will be.

Step 1. The first table is for women, the second is for men. Select the table appropriate for you and look it over. Calories are listed according to your target weight and for four different levels of physical activity. The number of fat grams you will consume is included in parentheses.

Step 2. Select your target weight as instructed. If you are over 30 years of age, round your target weight down to a weight included in the table. This means if you are 31 years old or older and your target weight is 127, you would round down to 120. Rounding down will help compensate for the gradual reduction in metabolic rate that occurs with aging. If you are 30

Women's Daily Caloric Intake (Fat Grams)

TARGET WEIGHT	COUCH POTATO	MILD ACTIVITY	MODERATE ACTIVITY	HEAVY ACTIVITY
100	1410 (23)	1570 (26)	1880 (31)	2190 (37)
110	1460 (24)	1620 (27)	1940 (32)	2270 (38)
120	1510 (25)	1670 (28)	2010 (33)	2340 (39)
130	1560 (26)	1730 (29)	2070 (34)	2420 (40)
140	1610 (27)	1790 (30)	2150 (36)	2510 (42)
150	1650 (28)	1840 (31)	2200 (37)	2570 (43)
160	1710 (29)	1900 (32)	2280 (38)	2660 (44)
170	1760 (30)	1960 (33)	2350 (39)	2740 (46)
180	1800 (31)	2000 (34)	2400 (40)	2800 (47)
190	1850 (32)	2050 (35)	2460 (41)	2870 (48)
200	1890 (33)	2090 (36)	2510 (42)	2930 (49)

HEIGHT	CORRECTION FACTOR	HEIGHT	CORRECTION FACTOR
4'9"	.93	5'5"	1.00
4'10"	.94	5'6"	1.01
4'11"	.95	5'7"	1.04
5'0"	.96	5'8"	1.05
5'1"	.97	5'9"	1.06
5'2"	.98	5'10"	1.07
5'3"	.99	5'11"	1.08
5'4"	1.00	6'0"	1.09

Men's Daily Caloric Intake (Fat Grams)

TARGET WEIGHT	COUCH POTATO	MILD ACTIVITY	MODERATE ACTIVITY	HEAVY ACTIVITY
120	1640 (27)	1820 (30)	2180 (36)	2550 (43)
130	1700 (28)	1890 (31)	2260 (38)	2640 (44)
140	1760 (29)	1950 (32)	2340 (39)	2740 (46)
150	1820 (30)	2020 (33)	2420 (40)	2830 (47)
160	1860 (31)	2070 (34)	2480 (41)	2890 (48)
170	1910 (32)	2120 (35)	2540 (42)	2970 (49)
180	1960 (33)	2180 (36)	2610 (43)	3040 (51)
190	2000 (34)	2220 (37)	2660 (44)	3110 (52)
200	2040 (35)	2260 (38)	2720 (45)	3170 (53)
210	2100 (36)	2330 (39)	2800 (46)	3260 (54)
220	2140 (37)	2380 (40)	2850 (47)	3320 (55)
230	2180 (38)	2420 (41)	2900 (48)	3390 (56)
240	2210 (39)	2450 (42)	2940 (49)	3430 (57)

HEIGHT	CORRECTION FACTOR	HEIGHT	CORRECTION FACTOR
5'0"	.90	5'9"	1.00
5'1"	.91	5'10"	1.01
5'2"	.92	5'11"	1.02
5'3"	.93	6'0"	1.03
5'4"	.94	6'1"	1.04
5'5"	.95	6'2"	1.06
5'6"	.97	6'3"	1.07
5'7"	.98	6'4"	1.08
5'8"	.99	6'5"	1.09

years of age or below, round to the nearest weight (127 would round to 130, for example, and 124 would round to 120).

Remember, your target weight should be no more than 40 pounds lower than your present weight. Find your target weight in column 1 of the appropriate caloric intake table and circle it. Now move on to Step 3.

Step 3. As you can see from these tables, in order to select your daily caloric intake (and fat grams), you must determine your approximate level of daily physical activity. You have done this already in chapter 10. Use that choice here and move across the table to the physical activity level appropriate for you.

Example: According to the table for women, a couch potato with a target weight of 130 pounds would require a daily intake of 1,560 calories and 26 grams of fat. Someone with the same weight, but a higher activity level (Mild Activity) would require 1,730 calories and 29 grams of fat.

Step 4. It is necessary to correct caloric intake and fat grams for height, using the correction factors at the bottom of the table you use. This step is important to those who are at the extremes, either very short or very tall, because, at a given weight, the taller person will have a greater skin surface area and a greater metabolic rate. The tables are based on average heights for women (5'4") and men (5'9"), and therefore the closer your height is to average, the smaller the correction will be.

Example: If the woman in the above example (Step 4) were 5'2" tall, it would be necessary to use the correction factor .98. (Find the .98 correction factor in the table next to 5'2".) Thus, you would multiply:

1560 x .98 = 1528 calories
26 fat grams x .98 = 25 grams of fat

This, of course, is not much of a change because this woman's height was close to average.

The following is a simple fill-in-the-blanks worksheet for you to follow. This one has been filled out as if by a thirty-five-year-old woman to show you how determining your daily caloric intake and fat grams works. You will use the worksheet on the next page.

Sample Caloric Intake and Fat Grams Worksheet

Fill in the blanks with your personal information.

1. Your current weight: __156 lbs__

2. Your target weight: __138 lbs (round down to 130)__

3. Your physical activity level: __Couch Potato__

4. Your uncorrected daily caloric intake: __1560 kcals__

5. Your uncorrected daily fat grams: __26 grams__

6. Your height: __5'9"__

7. Your height correction factor: __1.06__

8. Your corrected daily caloric intake:
   Multiply line #4 __1560__ x line #7 __1.06__ = __1654__

9. Your corrected daily fat grams:
   Multiply line #5 __26__ x line # 7 __1.06__ = __27.6 (round to 28)__

Caloric Intake and Fat Grams Worksheet

Fill in the blanks with your personal information.

1. Your current weight: _____

2. Your target weight: _____

3. Your physical activity level: _____

4. Your uncorrected daily caloric intake: _____

5. Your uncorrected daily fat grams: _____

6. Your height: _____

7. Your height correction factor: _____

8. Your corrected daily caloric intake:
   Multiply line #4 _____ x line #7 _____ = _____

9. Your corrected daily fat grams:
   Multiply line #5 _____ x line # 7 _____ = _____

You will use your corrected daily caloric intake and your corrected daily fat grams in the Jack Sprat plan. The next chapter will tell you how.

13

Target Menus

We have prepared two 28-day target menus to help you reach your (desired) target weight and to improve your health profile. The menus contain 1,700 and 2,400 daily calories. We chose these two levels because 1,700 represents the upper end of a typical maintenance diet for women and 2,400 represents the upper end of a typical maintenance diet for men.

Obviously, we don't expect your target daily caloric intake to fall exactly on 1,700 or 2,400 calories. They are merely convenient reference points. We have constructed each daily menu so that it can be altered easily. And because each of our menu tracts was strategically selected to take advantage of population clusters, the menus will require minuscule alterations to meet your individual needs. Here's an example.

Let's assume you are a 5'4", 150-pound female couch potato and that your target weight is 130 pounds. From the table you determined that you need 1,560 calories per day in order to sustain your target body weight of 130 pounds and your daily fat gram intake should be no greater than 26 grams. Obviously, we couldn't put together a 28-day plan for every possible caloric requirement, and this includes 1,560. Instead, we did the next best thing.

The Target 1700 menu is conveniently close to 1,560. All you have to do to individualize Day 1 of the menus is shave off 140 calories and 6 grams of fat per day. In anticipation of this need, we listed each food by calories and fat grams. Simply drop an item here and there to reach the desired levels.

Here's how it works.

Turn to Day 1 on the Target 1700 menus. In order to shave 140 calories from that day, all you would have to do is eat one-half of a brownie instead of a whole one (saving 65 calories and 1 gram of fat) and eliminate the one-half tablespoon of margarine (saving 50 calories and 5.7 grams of fat). It's that simple. You may have other ideas. That's fine, as long as you don't deviate from your goals for daily caloric intake and fat grams. Bear in mind that fat grams are the most important consideration. Therefore, when in doubt, make choices that help you keep fat gram intake at prescribed levels for that day, even if the calories are not exactly right.

In some cases, you will have the option of adding items to the menus instead of subtracting. If, for example, you are a large male with a target weight that requires 2,740 calories, you would need to add 340 calories to Day 1 of the Target 2400 menu. The best way to do this is by increasing portion sizes of items already on the menu. Adding two extra oat bran muffins would add 358 calories, for example, while adding only 3.6 grams of fat. Each day the menus offer different choices, so your decision could vary from day to day.

What if you don't want to fool around with altering the menus?

No problem. Even though it's simple, if you would rather not alter the menus, you have another option. Simply burn off excess calories and fat grams with mild postmeal exercise as described in chapter 11. Base the amount of time you need to exercise after meals on the number of calories and fat grams you need to burn off. It would be easy to burn off 140 calories and 6 grams of fat, for example, with brief walks after lunch and dinner.

Another option, of course, is using a combination of exercise and menu alterations, adjusting your choices daily as the menus change.

In putting the Jack Sprat plan together, we sought to provide a high degree of flexibility while taking you through step by step. As you can see, within the framework presented, options abound. All you have to do is determine which approach is easiest and most effective for you.

What if you do not have a "follower" personality, and, despite the options, you don't want to be bound by the Jack Sprat plan?

We have given you all the information you need to strike out on your own, and we encourage you to do so eventually. Certainly, you can pick and choose in bits and pieces from the daily menus within a tract that is right for you. You also can tap into the substitution tables. But we encourage you to take this approach *after* you graduate from the 28-day plan. You owe it to yourself to solidify your habits before going it alone.

The Jack Sprat plan was designed to be a lifelong investment. Other diets promote quick weight loss, but they don't take into account the body's overall dietary needs. The creators of such diets are smart enough to know they don't have to, because you won't be on the diet long enough for it to matter.

It was not simple putting together 28 days of menus on two separate tracts that meet target caloric and fat gram goals, while at the same time satisfying RDAs (Recommended Daily Allowances) for vitamins and minerals, meeting the body's need for fiber, and keeping sodium intake low (see mini-chapters on "Healthy Eating"). But we did it. We had to, because we know you will be eating like Jack Sprat for the rest of your life, and we want you to be not only lean but healthy as well.

Obviously, the challenge was greatest at the lowest caloric intakes (1,700 calories per day), especially when it comes to getting enough fiber. The target fiber content for each day on the Jack Sprat plan is 20 to 35 grams—an amount recommended by the American Dietetic Association and an amount far in excess of the average daily fiber intake of Americans. We generally eat too little fiber, and we pay for it with constipation, diverticulosis, and other gastrointestinal disorders. Lack of fiber also is thought to be an important factor in colon cancer.

Your sodium intake on the Jack Sprat plan will be limited, on average, to less than 3,000 mg per day, which is substantially less than the average sodium intake of Americans (4,000-8,000 mg/day). We have limited the use of processed foods as a means of keeping the sodium content low.

We have emphasized vegetables in the Jack Sprat diet without letting them take over your life. Although you will be eating lots of veggies, you won't find yourself telling bad rabbit jokes or complaining about eating nothing but cardboard and bean sprouts. The veggies you get will be all types, sizes, and colors. The main leafy green we emphasize is spinach. It's easy to come by, and it fits well into a number of Jack Sprat recipes. Other green veggies we emphasize include broccoli, asparagus, brussels sprouts, peas, green beans, lima beans, and green peppers. You'll also get lots of carrots, cauliflower, cabbage, eggplant, zucchini and summer squash, black-eyed peas, lentils, kidney beans, and, of course, potatoes. The good news is, we'll give you veggies without your realizing how much you are getting. And in the process, your body will thank you and reward you with increased health and decreased fatness.

Pasta shows up quite frequently, to everyone's delight. Pasta, the much maligned starch of the past, is today's star. We offer a number of pasta recipes and encourage you to create your own.

And don't think that we expect you to abandon all the things you have enjoyed throughout life. The menus contain steak, chicken, turkey, fish, pizza, even pork chops. You won't get a lot of them, but when you do you'll really appreciate it. And who knows, eventually your craving for such things may diminish to the point that you won't need them at all. When that day comes, you'll know you've arrived.

Some Helpful Hints for Using the Jack Sprat Menus

1. Before getting started, remember to determine the number of daily calories (and grams of fat) you need for your *desired* weight. (See tables on pages 63 and 64.)

2. To get started, choose either the 1,700- or the 2,400-calorie menu, whichever one is closest to the number of calories you need.

3. When adjusting the menus to fit your exact caloric needs, be certain to make changes that do not reduce the nutritional value of the diet. Reduce calories by eliminating desserts and snack items only. If you need to add calories to a menu (for example, increase the 1,700-calorie menu to, say, 1,920 calories) increase portion sizes and servings of nutritional items only—not desserts and snack items.

4. If a recipe on a daily menu is not to your liking, you can substitute for it with choices from the substitution tables (Resource 2). Be certain to choose only foods with similar fat gram content as the ones you are replacing. If possible, try to match up the caloric content too. But the calories are not as important as the fat grams.

5. If you cannot find the brands of foods listed in the menus, choose an alternative brand that is similar in fat grams and calories.

6. Popcorn is included as a snack on several menus. Generally, a 3-cup portion is recommended. To give you an idea of volume, there are 12 cups of popcorn in most microwave bags.

7. Yogurt is included in many menus. It's quick, easy, nutritious, and fat-free. It's also a good source of calcium. But if you feel the need to skip the yogurt in favor of something else, here are some suggestions:

> 1 cup of skim milk (86 calories)
> ½ cup of fat-free cottage cheese (70 calories)
> 1 slice Borden fat-free cheese (40 calories per slice) *and* 6 Snackwell Classic Golden Crackers (60 calories, 1 gram of fat)
> 2 ounces of fat-free cream cheese (50 calories) *and* 6 Snackwell Classic Golden Crackers (60 calories, 1 gram of fat)

8. The menus contain brands with which we are familiar. Some brands may not be available in your area. Feel free to choose other brands. Match labels and make certain your brand contains similar caloric and fat gram values.

9. Don't make assumptions. There can be a wide range of fat gram and caloric values on "low-fat" products. "Low-fat" milk (2 percent), for example, is actually 37.5 percent fat by calories and contains 5 grams of fat per serving. Read the labels carefully.

10. In lower calorie diets it is difficult to make certain all essential vitamins and trace minerals are included. It is difficult to get sufficient vitamin D, for example, if you don't drink enough skim milk. For this reason, we recommend taking a good multivitamin/mineral tablet each day.

11. The fat grams and calories vary slightly for Healthy Choice ice cream. You can choose a flavor you prefer and adjust the menu accordingly.

12. You can use either egg whites or egg substitute in recipes unless one is specified. For instance, use only egg whites in the pound cake and egg substitute when making scrambled eggs.

14

The Grocery List

Select the target level (1700 or 2400) that is right for you. Read over the menus to acquaint yourself with the foods you will eat that week. Then turn to the grocery list. This is a "real" grocery list: take it to the store and check off items as you go.

While you shop, you might find it interesting to take note of how supermarkets are organized. Here's the lowdown.

1. Dairy products are placed in the least convenient corner of the building. This is because almost everyone who enters is going to buy milk, and it makes good business sense to make customers walk past all the other food items on their way there. For this reason, it's a good idea not to shop when you are hungry The power of suggestion and the design of the market can influence you to buy lots of things you hadn't planned on. And if your hunger is strong, chances are you'll emerge with a cart full of high-fat, high-calorie goodies.

2. Meats, poultry, and seafood are placed along the rear wall of the store so that no matter which aisle you enter, you are looking in that direction. This is important to the store, because the meat counter is the most profitable section.

3. Produce generally greets you soon after you enter, and you almost always have to walk through that section on the way

to somewhere else. Produce offers an attractive display that highly influences your feelings about the store. Shiny fruits and vegetables arranged in orderly stacks suggest high quality and tender loving care, and the appearance of the produce section may be one of the most important factors in your choice of where to shop for food.

4. In general, the most profitable items are situated around the perimeter of the store (meats, dairy, produce, deli, bakery). Offerings on the perimeter tend to be the most impressive and serve to distinguish one store from another.

5. Less profitable items are relegated to the interior of the store within the aisles. This is where you are likely to find your best buys. Cereals, which provide high profits, are the exception. To compensate, cereal gets its own aisle and plenty of space.

Q. What if I need to alter the menus to fit my exact caloric and fat gram needs? What if my caloric needs are 1,560, for instance, and the menus provide 1,700 calories? How will that affect the grocery list?

A. It won't. Regardless of your needs or the target menu you choose, the Jack Sprat plan is designed so that any alterations you make shouldn't be large enough to affect your choices at the supermarket. If, for example, as discussed in previous chapters, you were to alter your menu by eating one-half of a brownie instead of a whole one and by reducing your margarine intake by half, you would still purchase the brownie mix and the margarine in the same quantities.

Q. If I am buying for more than one person, what should I do?

A. The grocery list is constructed for one person, with the exception of recipe items, which are indicated by the recipe numbers. Since the recipes serve two or more people, you wouldn't have to increase these items; all you need to do is increase your purchases of the nonrecipe items.

Q. What if the wife's target is 1,700 and the husband's is 2,400? How will that affect the grocery list?

A. The recipes serve two to four, regardless of the target level, so that's not a problem. To make certain you have more than enough nonrecipe foods at home for both of you, and to simplify matters, we recommend that in this case you use the 2400 grocery list only and double the purchase of nonrecipe items. Doubling nonrecipe items will ensure that you have a sufficient number of apples, loaves of bread, containers of fat-free yogurt, and so forth. Bear in mind that many foods—a box of sourdough pretzels, a half-gallon of fat-free ice cream, a jar of applesauce—must be purchased in bulk and could last more than one week, or they can be used to serve the needs of more than one person. Decision making on such items will become second nature once you immerse yourself in the plan.

Q. **What happens if I live and eat alone and I buy foods that make a recipe for two or four?**

A. No problem. Put leftovers in the freezer and pull them out another day. You can fit leftovers into the Jack Sprat plan in any number of ways. One: substitute leftovers for lunches or future dinners, as long as the fat grams and calories match up reasonably well. Two: repeat a complete day's menu when you want to use the leftovers. This, in effect, expands the Jack Sprat plan. Each day you repeat within the 28-day cycle expands the cycle by one day. Keep in mind that there is nothing magical about the order of the daily menus. Our purpose was simply to give you lots of variety. Three: if you see that you are getting too many leftovers, cut the recipes down to suit your circumstances.

Before taking off for the supermarket, check the staples on the last page of the grocery list and compare with what you already have on the shelves at home. It's also a good idea to clear your home shelves of sludge. Get rid of the potato chips, salami, franks, and Twinkies, and make certain that from now on your food needs will be met with the Jack Sprat plan only. And remember, if you need to cheat, we'll show you how with the Jack Sprat "warthog" days. More on that later.

Q. **What if I don't like a recipe for a given day during the week?**

A. Examine the week's menus before you take the grocery list to the market. If you find foods you don't like, make note of the recipe number. This number corresponds with numbers on the grocery list. Simply delete items with this particular number from the list before you go shopping. Replace canceled foods with something you like. Check the substitution choices in Resource 2. When you find something you like that fits the parameters you require for calories and grams of fat, check out the recipe and add whatever is necessary to the grocery list.

Some items on the grocery list will be used in more than one recipe. If so, they will have more than one number beside them, indicating the various recipes in which they are to be used. Onions, for example, may be used in many different places. When canceling a recipe that contains onions, simply lower the amount purchased, but make certain to cover needs in other recipes. Most often, this won't be much of a consideration, because such items are purchased in batches, clumps, boxes, or some other bulk form.

Q. What if the wife wants to follow the Jack Sprat plan but the husband doesn't?

A. This is a common problem. Occasionally, it's the other way around—the husband wants to change—but that is extremely rare. Years ago we worked with Millie, a woman who desperately wanted to change the eating habits of her husband, Joe. And for good reason. In his early sixties, he was a wreck. He was at least 70 pounds overweight, his blood pressure was too high (despite medication), his blood sugar was out of control, and his cholesterol was well over 300 mg/dl.

But to spite Millie's good efforts on his behalf, Joe would sneak off and buy corn chips, cold cuts, and ice cream. There was no way she could win with her husband acting like a child. Finally, to save her sanity, we advised her to give up on him and start worrying about herself.

This was hard for Millie, the devoted wife, but eventually she began faithfully following a healthy low-fat diet and taking long walks on her own. She also quit nagging Joe and worrying about what he was eating. A few years went by before we saw Millie again. She looked like a different person. There was a spring in her step, and she had recaptured the figure of a young woman. When asked about Joe, she smiled and told us: "One day I got so mad at him sitting there eating a big bag of chips—right in front of me—I thought I'd explode. I told him if he was going to keep driving himself to ruin, he'd better make sure his life insurance premiums were paid up, because I sure didn't intend to sit around feeling sorry for myself after he was gone." She shrugged, then said: "That got to him. He was mad as a hornet at first, but then he started coming around. I think he knows there's life left in this old gal, and if he's smart he'll try to stay around to enjoy me."

We don't have any pat answers for convincing recalcitrant spouses or children to change. Your best bet is to do what you can for yourself. Make the Jack Sprat recipes and share them with your spouse. They're tasty and should be received well. But we are aware that there are hardcore sludge addicts who will refuse anything that smacks of health. If you are married to one, your best bet is to accept it. And learn from Millie. Nagging will get you nowhere. But check to see that life insurance premiums are paid up in full.

15

The 28-Day Plan

You are now ready to get started. When you turn to the target tract you have selected, you will find 28 days of menus, divided into four weeks. Look over the first week, then study the accompanying grocery list that provides everything you need.

At the end of the 28 days of menus, you will find four warthog alternative days from which you can choose when you have the need.

For recipes you will use during the 28-day plan, turn to Resource 1. Plan recipes are numbered chronologically from 1 to 52. The numbers appear on the menus *and* in Resources 1 and 2 for easy reference.

When you want to make substitutions in the 28-day plan, turn to Resource 2, the substitution tables. We also have included fast-food tables in Resource 3 from which you can select lunches and dinners.

When brainstorming about low-fat diets and strategies you will use when you graduate from the 28-day plan, consult Resource 4, "More Smart Choices." Here you will learn how substituting a tasty low-fat food for a high-fat food, or making substitutions in recipes, can save you fat grams.

Note: Although we have deemphasized calories in favor of

emphasizing fat intake, this does not mean that caloric intake is not important. If you take in too many calories, even on a low-fat diet, eventually you will gain weight. The number of pounds you gain will, of course, be much less than it would be on a high-fat diet, but it will occur nonetheless. For this reason, it is important that you tailor the daily menus as closely as possible to the number of calories we recommend to support your target weight (see chapter 12). In this way you will enhance your progress by getting the dual benefits of a low-fat diet combined with an appropriate daily caloric intake. Benefits will be further enhanced when you initiate a Jack Sprat Smart Exercise program.

After you get a good start in the plan, read part 3. You will learn more about body fat, healthy eating, and exercise. But there is no hurry. At this point, you should know everything you need to know to get you started and moving in the right direction.

Target 1700 Grocery List—Week 1

PRODUCE

___ Apples
___ Blueberries, fresh or frozen *#1*
___ Grapes

___ Pears (for Jell-O)
___ Bananas
___ Strawberries, fresh or frozen *#12*

___ Broccoli *#9, #13*
___ Mushrooms *#9, #10, #13*
___ Celery *#8*
___ Carrots *#9, #10, #13*
___ Cauliflower *#9, #10*
___ Zucchini *#13*
___ Romaine lettuce *#5*
___ Head lettuce *#10*
___ Potatoes

___ Onions *#9, #13*
___ Tomatoes *#10*
___ Cucumbers *#5*
___ Corn on the cob
___ Green pepper *#10*
___ Peas
___ Snow peas *#9*
___ Spinach *#4*
___ Garlic *#13*

GRAINS/PASTA/RICE

Make sure breads are fat-free.

___ Whole wheat bread
___ French bread
___ Whole wheat rolls
___ Spaghetti
___ Cereal (100% bran, ⅓ cup
    equals 70 calories and no
    more than 1.4 grams fat)

___ Cereal (with less than 1 gram
    fat per serving)
___ Brown rice *#9*
___ Jumbo pasta shells *#4*
___ Rigatoni or ziti *#5*
___ Fettucine *#13*

DAIRY/EGGS

___ Skim milk *#7, #12, #13*
___ Yoplait fat-free light yogurt
___ Buttermilk *#1, #6, #12*
___ Eggs or egg substitute *#1, #7,*
    #12
___ Light ricotta cheese *#4*

___ Fat-free mozzarella cheese *#4*
___ Low-fat cheddar cheese *#10*
___ Margarine
___ Fat-free sour cream
___ Fat-free plain yogurt *#3, #11*
___ Parmesan cheese *#4, #6, #13*

Note: Items to be used in recipes are followed by the recipe numbers from Resource 1.

MEAT/POULTRY/FISH

___ Lean sirloin steak
___ Chicken breasts *#6, #9*
___ Turkey breast *#10* and sliced
    turkey for sandwiches

___ Cod or other whitefish *#2*
___ Shrimp *#13*

JUICE/SNACKS/DESSERTS

___ Orange juice
___ Orville Redenbacher Smart-
    Pop popcorn
___ Snyder's sourdough pretzels
___ Betty Crocker low-fat brownie
    mix

___ Healthy Choice low-fat ice
    cream
___ Chocolate chip cookies (135
    calories each)
___ Sugar-free Jell-O

STAPLES

___ Molasses *#1*
___ Honey *#1, #3, #5, #7, #12*
___ Fat-free salad dressing *#3, #8*
___ Low-calorie or fat-free Italian
    dressing
___ Maple syrup *#11*
___ Lemon juice *#2, #3, #5*
___ Sweet pickle relish *#1, #8*
___ Low-sodium soy sauce *#9*
___ Dijon mustard *#8*

___ Vanilla *#7, #12*
___ Olive oil *#5*
___ All-purpose flour *#12*
___ Oat bran *#1, #12*
___ Whole wheat flour *#1, #12*
___ Baking soda *#1, #12*
___ Baking powder *#12*
___ Wheat germ *#12*
___ Poppyseeds *#11*

SPICES

___ Tarragon *#3*
___ Cajun seasoning *#13*
___ Basil *#5*

___ Salt
___ Pepper

MISCELLANEOUS

___ Salmon, canned *#5*
___ Water-packed tuna, canned *#8*
___ Quick-cooking tapioca *#7*

___ Pitted black olives *#5*
___ Fat-free spaghetti sauce *#4*
___ Unsweetened applesauce *#12*

Target 1700 Menu for Day 1 (Week 1)

	TOTAL FAT (GRAMS)	SATURATED FAT (GRAMS)	CALORIES
Breakfast			
Cold cereal (½ cup)	1.0	0.1	100
Bran cereal (⅓ cup)	1.4	0.3	70
Skim milk (1 cup)	0.4	0.3	86
Snack			
Yoplait fat-free light yogurt (6 ounces)	0.0	0.0	90
Lunch			
Wendy's grilled chicken sandwich (1)	7.0	1.5	290
Wendy's side salad (1)	3.0	0.0	60
Reduced-calorie Italian dressing (2 tablespoons)	3.0	0.0	40
Snack			
Oat bran muffin (1) *#1*	1.8	0.3	179
Dinner			
Broiled codfish (4 ounces) *#2*	1.0	0.2	118
Tartar sauce (2 tablespoons) *#3*	0.1	0.0	28
Potato, baked (1 medium)	0.2	0.1	220
Broccoli, steamed (1 cup)	0.4	0.1	46
French bread (1 slice)	1.0	0.2	70
Margarine (½ tablespoon)	5.7	1.0	50
Betty Crocker low-fat brownie (1)	2.5	0.5	130
Snack			
Snyder's sourdough pretzel (1)	0.0	0.0	111

Note: Recipe numbers follow dishes that appear in Resource 1.

Total fat: 28.5 grams (15%)   Saturated fat: 4.6 grams   Calories: 1689

Target 1700 Menu for Day 2 (Week 1)

	TOTAL FAT (GRAMS)	SATURATED FAT (GRAMS)	CALORIES
Breakfast			
Cold cereal (½ cup)	1.0	0.1	100
Bran cereal (⅓ cup)	1.4	0.3	70
Skim milk (1 cup)	0.4	0.3	86
Banana (1)	0.6	0.1	105
Snack			
Yoplait fat-free light yogurt (6 ounces)	0.0	0.0	90
Lunch			
Turkey sandwich:			
Turkey (w/o skin, 4 ounces)	2.7	0.8	133
Whole wheat bread (2 slices)	2.0	0.4	130
Lettuce (1 piece)	0.0	0.0	2
Tomato (2 slices)	0.1	0.0	8
Carrots, raw (2 medium)	0.3	0.0	62
Snack			
Oat bran muffin (1) *#1*	1.8	0.3	179
Apple (1)	0.5	0.1	81
Dinner			
Large stuffed pasta shells (3) *#4*	4.8	3.0	232
Tossed salad (2 cups)	0.2	0.0	20
Fat-free Italian dressing (2 tablespoons)	0.0	0.0	28
French bread (1 slice)	1.0	0.2	70
Margarine (½ tablespoon)	5.7	1.0	50
Betty Crocker low-fat brownie (1)	2.5	0.5	130
Snack			
Orville Redenbacher Smart-Pop popcorn (6 cups)	2.0	2.0	100

Note: Recipe numbers follow dishes that appear in Resource 1.

Total fat: 27.0 grams (14%)   *Saturated fat: 9.1 grams*   *Calories: 1676*

Target 1700 Menu for Day 3 (Week 1)

	TOTAL FAT (GRAMS)	SATURATED FAT (GRAMS)	CALORIES
Breakfast			
Cold cereal (½ cup)	1.0	0.1	100
Bran cereal (⅓ cup)	1.4	0.3	70
Skim milk (1 cup)	0.4	0.3	86
Banana (1)	0.6	0.1	105
Snack			
Grapes (20)	0.2	0.0	72
Lunch			
Salmon salad (1½ cups) #5	9.7	0.8	310
French bread (1 slice)	1.0	0.2	70
Chocolate chip cookie (1)	6.0	1.9	135
Snack			
Yoplait fat-free light yogurt (6 ounces)	0.0	0.0	90
Dinner			
Parmesan chicken (1 serving) #6	5.7	2.6	199
Brown rice (¾ cup)	1.0	0.0	180
Peas and carrots (½ cup each)	0.3	0.1	69
Whole wheat bread (1 slice)	1.0	0.2	65
Tapioca pudding (1 cup) #7	0.4	0.3	183
Snack			
Sugar-free Jell-O (1 cup, ½ pear)	0.0	0.0	54

Note: Recipe numbers follow dishes that appear in Resource 1.

Total fat: 28.7 grams (14%)   Saturated fat: 6.9 grams   Calories: 1788

Target 1700 Menu for Day 4 (Week 1)

	TOTAL FAT (GRAMS)	SATURATED FAT (GRAMS)	CALORIES
Breakfast			
Cold cereal (½ cup)	1.0	0.1	100
Skim milk (1 cup)	0.4	0.3	86
Banana (1)	0.6	0.1	105
Bran cereal (⅓ cup)	1.4	0.3	70
Snack			
Oat bran muffin (1) *#1*	1.8	0.3	179
Lunch			
McDonald's McLean Deluxe (1)	12.0	4.0	340
McDonald's low-fat hot fudge sundae (1)	5.0	2.4	290
Snack			
Apple (1)	0.5	0.1	81
Dinner			
Spaghetti with sauce (no meat):			
Spaghetti, cooked (1 cup)	1.0	0.1	210
Fat-free spaghetti sauce (½ cup)	0.0	0.8	94
French bread (1 slice)	1.0	0.2	70
Tossed salad (2 cups)	0.4	0.1	41
Fat-free Italian dressing (2 tablespoons)	0.0	0.0	28
Snack			
Snyder's sourdough pretzel (1)	0.0	0.0	111

Note: Recipe numbers follow dishes that appear in Resource 1.

Total fat: 25.1 grams (12%)   Saturated fat: 8.8 grams   Calories: 1805

Target 1700 Menu for Day 5 (Week 1)

	TOTAL FAT (GRAMS)	SATURATED FAT (GRAMS)	CALORIES
Breakfast			
McDonald's hotcakes with syrup only (1 order)	4.0	3.7	360
Orange juice (6 ounces)	0.0	0.0	80
Snack			
Grapes (10)	0.1	0.0	36
Lunch			
Tuna sandwich:			
Tuna salad (1 serving) #8	2.7	0.6	171
Whole wheat bread (2 slices)	2.0	0.4	130
Carrots, raw (2 medium)	0.3	0.0	62
Snack			
Banana (1)	0.6	0.1	105
Skim milk (1 cup)	0.8	0.6	86
Dinner			
Stir-fry vegetables with chicken (1 serving) #9	11.0	2.1	261
Brown rice (½ cup)	1.0	0.0	120
Sugar-free Jell-O (1 cup, ½ pear)	0.0	0.0	54
Skim milk (1 cup)	0.4	0.3	86
Snack			
Healthy Choice low-fat ice cream (½ cup)	2.0	1.0	120
Wheat germ (2 tablespoons)	1.0	0.0	50

Note: Recipe numbers follow dishes that appear in Resource 1.

Total fat: 25.9 grams (14%)   *Saturated fat: 8.8 grams*   *Calories: 1721*

Target 1700 Menu for Day 6 (Week 1)

	TOTAL FAT (GRAMS)	SATURATED FAT (GRAMS)	CALORIES
Breakfast			
Cold cereal (½ cup)	1.0	0.1	100
Banana (1)	0.6	0.1	105
Skim milk (½ cup)	0.2	0.1	43
Snack			
Oat bran muffin (1) *#1*	1.8	0.3	179
Skim milk (1 cup)	0.4	0.3	86
Lunch			
Chef salad (2 cups) *#10*	7.0	3.9	156
Poppyseed dressing (¼ cup) *#11*	0.2	0.0	54
Whole wheat roll (1)	3.4	0.8	52
Snack			
Apple (1)	0.5	0.1	81
Dinner			
Lean sirloin steak, broiled (4-ounce serving)	8.0	3.1	239
Potato, baked (1 medium)	0.2	0.1	220
Fat-free sour cream (4 tablespoons)	0.0	0.0	60
Peas (½ cup)	0.2	0.0	34
Corn on the cob (1 ear)	1.1	0.2	77
French bread (1 slice)	1.0	0.2	70
Betty Crocker low-fat brownie (1)	2.5	0.5	130
Snack			
Sugar-free Jell-O (1 cup, ½ pear)	0.0	0.0	54

Note: Recipe numbers follow dishes that appear in Resource 1.

Total fat: 28.1 grams (14%)   Saturated fat: 9.8 grams   Calories: 1740

Target 1700 Menu for Day 7 (Week 1)

	TOTAL FAT (GRAMS)	SATURATED FAT (GRAMS)	CALORIES
Breakfast			
Multi-grain pancakes *#12* (2 medium size)	8.0	1.6	323
Strawberries, sliced (1 cup)	0.6	0.0	45
Orange juice (1 cup)	0.1	0.0	110
Snack			
Yoplait fat-free light yogurt (6 ounces)	0.0	0.0	90
Lunch			
Tuna sandwich:			
Tuna salad (1 serving) *#8*	2.7	0.6	171
Whole wheat bread (2 slices)	2.0	0.4	130
Carrots, raw (2 medium)	0.3	0.0	62
Snack			
Oat bran muffin *(1) #1*	1.8	0.3	179
Skim milk (1 cup)	0.4	0.3	86
Dinner			
Shrimp fettucine (1 serving) *#13*	7.1	3.2	425
Spinach (½ cup)	0.2	0.0	21
French bread (1 slice)	1.0	0.2	70
Snack			
Orville Redenbacher Smart-Pop popcorn (3 cups)	1.0	1.0	50

Note: Recipe numbers follow dishes that appear in Resource 1.

Total fat: 25.2 grams (13%)   Saturated fat: 7.6 grams   Calories: 1762

Target 1700 Grocery List—Week 2

PRODUCE

___ Grapefruit
___ Cantaloupe
___ Apples
___ Seedless raisins
___ Grapes

___ Bananas
___ Orange
___ Pears
___ Strawberries

___ Broccoli *#20, #22*
___ Mushrooms *#10, #22, #25*
___ Celery *#14*
___ Carrots *#10*
___ Cauliflower *#10*
___ Zucchini *#18, #24*
___ Summer squash
___ Head lettuce *#10*
___ Potatoes *#18, #21, #23*
___ Onions *#14, #18, #20, #21,*
    #22, #23, #24

___ Tomatoes *#10, #18, #24*
___ Cucumber *#17*
___ Corn on the cob
___ Green pepper *#10, #14, #18, #24*
___ Green beans
___ Eggplant *#18, #26*
___ Spinach *#22, #25*
___ Garlic *#14, #21, #22, #26*
___ Asparagus
___ Scallions *#17*
___ Sprouts *#24*

GRAINS/PASTA/RICE

Make sure breads are fat-free.
___ Whole wheat bread
___ Sourdough bread
___ French bread
___ Oatmeal
___ English muffins
___ Whole wheat lasagna noodles
    #22, #25
___ Bagels

___ Rice cakes
___ Pita pockets *#24*
___ Ziti *#26*
___ Cereal (100% bran, ⅓ cup
    equals 70 calories and no
    more than 1.4 grams fat)
___ Cereal (with less than 1 gram
    fat per serving)
___ Brown rice *#14, #17, #20*

DAIRY/EGGS

___ Skim milk *#7, #15*
___ Yoplait fat-free light yogurt
___ Healthy Choice egg substitute
    (for scrambled eggs)
___ Eggs (or egg substitute) *#7, #25*
___ Fat-free cheese slices *#19, #24*
___ Fat-free mozzarella cheese *#22*

___ Low-fat cheddar cheese *#10, #15*
___ Parmesan cheese *#20, #22, #26*
___ Fat-free cottage cheese *#20,*
    #25, #26
___ Margarine *#19*
___ Fat-free sour cream
___ Fat-free plain yogurt *#11*

Note: Items to be used in recipes are followed by the recipe numbers from Resource 1.

MEAT/POULTRY/FISH

___ Chicken breasts #16, #21   ___ Turkey breast #10

JUICE/SNACKS/DESSERTS

___ Orange juice
___ Orville Redenbacher Smart-
      Pop popcorn
___ Snyder's sourdough pretzels
___ Betty Crocker low-fat brownie
      mix

___ Healthy Choice low-fat ice
      cream
___ Chocolate syrup
___ Fat-free hot fudge sauce
___ Sugar-free chocolate pudding

STAPLES

___ Honey #7, #16
___ Maple syrup #11
___ Poppyseeds #11
___ Lemon juice #16, #17
___ Dijon mustard #16, #24

___ Olive oil #17, #18
___ All-purpose flour #15, #23
___ Vinegar #17, #18
___ Wheat germ
___ Fruit spread (no sugar added)

SPICES

___ Marjoram #23
___ Oregano #14, #17, #21, #26
___ Parsley #18, #22, #23, #26
___ Cumin #21
___ Cayenne pepper #14, #15
___ Paprika #15

___ Thyme #23
___ Chives #15
___ Basil #18, #26
___ Chili powder #21
___ Salt
___ Pepper

MISCELLANEOUS

___ Red beans, canned #14
___ Green chilies, canned #21
___ Dried lentils #17
___ Tomatoes, canned #17
___ Garbanzo beans, canned #18
___ Dry white beans #21
___ Quick-cooking tapioca #7

___ Fat-free spaghetti sauce #22,
      #25, #26
___ Unsweetened applesauce #12
___ Unsalted pecans
___ Fat-free saltine crackers
___ Peanut butter
___ Corn, canned

Target 1700 Menu for Day 8 (Week 2)

	TOTAL FAT (GRAMS)	SATURATED FAT (GRAMS)	CALORIES
Breakfast			
Oatmeal, cooked (1 cup)	2.0	0.4	145
Orange juice (1 cup)	0.1	0.0	110
Skim milk (1 cup)	0.4	0.3	86
Snack			
Grapes (20)	0.2	0.0	72
Lunch			
Taco Bell lite soft taco supreme (1)	5.0	2.0	199
Taco bell cinnamon twists (1 order)	6.0	3.0	139
Snack			
Orville Redenbacher Smart-Pop popcorn (6 cups)	2.0	2.0	100
Dinner			
Red beans and rice (1 serving) *#14*	1.7	0.3	229
Broccoli, cooked (1 cup)	0.4	0.1	46
Low-fat cheese sauce (½ cup) *#15*	2.4	1.4	121
Tomato (3 slices)	0.2	0.0	12
Carrots, cooked (½ cup)	0.1	0.0	35
Sugar-free chocolate pudding (1 cup)	1.0	0.0	130
Snack			
Snyder's sourdough pretzels (2)	0.0	0.0	222

Note: Recipe numbers follow dishes that appear in Resource 1.

Total fat: 21.5 grams (12%)   Saturated fat: 9.5 grams   Calories: 1646

Target 1700 Menu for Day 9 (Week 2)

	TOTAL FAT (GRAMS)	SATURATED FAT (GRAMS)	CALORIES
Breakfast			
English muffin (1)	1.0	0.3	140
Fruit spread (2 tablespoons)	0.0	0.0	84
Cantaloupe (½)	0.7	0.1	94
Skim milk (1 cup)	0.4	0.3	86
Snack			
Yoplait fat-free light yogurt (6 ounces)	0.0	0.0	90
Lunch			
Chef salad (2 cups) *#10*	7.0	3.9	156
Poppyseed dressing (¼ cup) *#11*	0.2	0.0	54
Whole wheat bread (2 slices)	2.0	0.4	130
Snack			
Apple (1)	0.5	0.1	81
Rice cake (1)	0.0	0.0	35
Dinner			
Chicken with Dijon mustard (1 serving) *#16*	4.9	0.9	205
Lentil salad (1 cup) *#17*	0.6	0.1	65
Asparagus, cooked (1 cup)	0.6	0.2	44
Skim milk (1 cup)	0.4	0.3	86
Snack			
Healthy Choice low-fat ice cream (½ cup)	2.0	1.0	120
Chocolate syrup (2 tablespoons)	1.0	0.4	92
Unsalted pecans (about 8)	9.0	0.8	93
Wheat germ (2 tablespoons)	1.0	0.0	50

Note: Recipe numbers follow dishes that appear in Resource 1.

Total fat: 31.3 grams (17%)   Saturated fat: 8.8 grams   Calories: 1705

Target 1700 Menu for Day 10 (Week 2)

	TOTAL FAT (GRAMS)	SATURATED FAT (GRAMS)	CALORIES
Breakfast			
Cold cereal (½ cup)	1.0	0.1	100
Bran cereal (⅓ cup)	1.4	0.3	70
Strawberries (½ cup)	0.3	0.0	22
Skim milk (1 cup)	0.4	0.3	86
Snack			
Yoplait fat-free light yogurt (6 ounces)	0.0	0.0	90
Lunch			
McDonald's chunky chicken salad (1)	5.0	1.1	160
Reduced-calorie French dressing (1 packet)	8.0	1.0	160
McDonald's low-fat hot fudge sundae (1)	5.0	2.4	290
Snack			
Apple (1)	0.5	0.1	81
Dinner			
Grilled skinless chicken breast (1)	7.6	2.2	193
Vegetable medley (1 serving) *#18*	4.2	0.5	126
French bread (1 slice)	1.0	0.2	70
Snack			
Bagel (1)	1.5	0.2	185
Fruit spread (1 tablespoon)	0.0	0.0	42
Skim milk (1 cup)	0.4	0.3	86

Note: Recipe numbers follow dishes that appear in Resource 1.

Total fat: 36.3 grams (19%)   Saturated fat: 8.7 grams   Calories: 1761

Target 1700 Menu for Day 11
(Week 2)

	TOTAL FAT (GRAMS)	SATURATED FAT (GRAMS)	CALORIES
Breakfast			
Oatmeal, cooked (1 cup)	2.0	0.4	145
Banana (1)	0.6	0.1	105
Skim milk (1 cup)	0.4	0.3	86
Snack			
Yoplait fat-free light yogurt (6 ounces)	0.0	0.0	90
Lunch			
Grilled cheese (1) *#19*	8.0	1.6	260
Tomato (2 slices)	0.1	0.0	8
Carrots, raw (½ cup)	0.1	0.0	24
Pear (1)	0.7	0.0	98
Snack			
Orville Redenbacher Smart-Pop popcorn (6 cups)	2.0	2.0	100
Dinner			
Broccoli-rice casserole (1 serving) *#20*	5.3	2.9	221
Summer squash, cooked (1 cup)	0.6	0.1	36
Whole wheat bread (2 slices)	2.0	0.4	130
Betty Crocker low-fat brownie (1)	2.5	0.5	130
Skim milk (1 cup)	0.4	0.3	86
Snack			
Snyder's sourdough pretzel (1)	0.0	0.0	111

Note: Recipe numbers follow dishes that appear in Resource 1.

Total fat: 24.7 grams (14%)   Saturated fat: 8.6 grams   Calories: 1630

Target 1700 Menu for Day 12
(Week 2)

	TOTAL FAT (GRAMS)	SATURATED FAT (GRAMS)	CALORIES
Breakfast			
Healthy Choice egg substitute, scrambled (½ cup)	0.0	0.0	50
Whole wheat bread (2 slices)	2.0	0.4	130
Margarine (½ tablespoon)	5.7	1.0	50
Fruit spread (2 tablespoons)	0.0	0.0	84
Unsweetened applesauce (¼ cup)	0.1	0.0	26
Skim milk (1 cup)	0.4	0.3	86
Snack			
Apple (1)	0.5	0.1	81
Lunch			
White bean chili (1 serving) #21	2.9	0.7	235
Fat-free saltine crackers (5)	0.0	0.0	50
Snack			
Banana (1)	0.6	0.1	105
Dinner			
Vegetable lasagna (1 serving) #22	6.9	3.6	300
Green beans (1 cup)	0.2	0.0	50
Corn, canned (½ cup)	1.1	0.2	89
French bread (2 slices)	1.0	0.2	140
Sugar-free chocolate pudding (1 cup)	1.0	0.0	130
Snack			
Orville Redenbacher Smart-Pop popcorn (6 cups)	2.0	2.0	100

Note: Recipe numbers follow dishes that appear in Resource 1.

Total fat: 28.4 grams (15%)   Saturated fat: 9.8 grams   Calories: 1706

Target 1700 Menu for Day 13
(Week 2)

	TOTAL FAT (GRAMS)	SATURATED FAT (GRAMS)	CALORIES
Breakfast			
Bagel (1)	1.5	0.2	185
Margarine (½ tablespoon)	5.7	1.0	50
Fruit spread (2 tablespoons)	0.0	0.0	84
Grapefruit (½)	0.1	0.0	38
Snack			
Peanut butter and crackers:			
4 saltines and 2 tablespoons peanut butter	18.0	3.3	221
Orange (1)	0.0	0.0	62
Skim milk (1 cup)	0.4	0.3	86
Lunch			
Potato soup (1 serving) *#23*	0.4	0.2	133
Pita with veggies (1) *#24*	2.2	0.1	209
Snack			
Pear (1)	0.7	0.0	98
Dinner			
Spinach mushroom lasagna (1 serving) *#25*	1.0	0.0	235
Tossed salad (2 cups)	0.2	0.0	41
Poppyseed dressing (1 serving) *#11*	0.2	0.0	54
Sourdough bread (1 slice)	0.5	0.0	68
Snack			
Healthy Choice low-fat ice cream (½ cup)	2.0	1.0	120
Fat-free hot fudge sauce (1 tablespoons)	0.0	0.0	45
Wheat germ (2 tablespoons)	1.0	0.0	50

Note: Recipe numbers follow dishes that appear in Resource 1.

Total fat: 33.9 grams (17%)   Saturated fat: 6.1 grams   Calories: 1779

Target 1700 Menu for Day 14 (Week 2)

	TOTAL FAT (GRAMS)	SATURATED FAT (GRAMS)	CALORIES
Breakfast			
Cold cereal (½ cup)	1.0	0.1	100
Wheat germ (2 tablespoons)	1.0	0.0	50
Skim milk (1 cup)	0.4	0.3	86
Seedless raisins (¼ cup)	0.3	0.1	108
Orange juice (1 cup)	0.4	0.0	110
Snack			
Banana (1)	0.6	0.1	105
Lunch			
Potato, baked (1 medium)	0.2	0.1	220
Fat-free sour cream (4 tablespoons)	0.0	0.0	60
Carrots, raw or steamed (½ cup)	0.1	0.0	24
Broccoli, raw or steamed (½ cup)	0.2	0.0	12
Snack			
Cantaloupe (½)	0.7	0.1	94
Dinner			
Eggplant Parmesan with pasta (1 serving) #26	6.9	3.7	300
Corn on the cob (1 ear)	1.1	0.2	77
Tapioca pudding (1 cup) #7	0.4	0.3	183
Snack			
Orville Redenbacher Smart-Pop popcorn (6 cups)	2.0	2.0	100

Note: Recipe numbers follow dishes that appear in Resource 1.

Total fat: 15.3 grams (8%)   *Saturated fat: 7.0 grams*   *Calories: 1629*

Target 1700 Grocery List—Week 3

PRODUCE

___ Oranges
___ Granny Smith apples *#51*
___ Apples (for snacks)
___ Blueberries, fresh or frozen *#33*
___ Bananas

___ Strawberries, fresh or frozen *#12*
___ Grapefruit
___ Lemons
___ Seedless raisins *#30, #31, #51*
___ Nectarines

___ Broccoli
___ Mushrooms *#37, #52*
___ Celery *#3, #28*
___ Carrots *#31, #37*
___ Cauliflower
___ Zucchini *#24, #38, #52*
___ Potatoes *#23, #28, #29*
___ Onions *#23, #24, #28, #38*

___ Tomatoes *#24, #36, #38*
___ Green beans *#36*
___ Corn on the cob
___ Green pepper *#24, #38*
___ Spinach *#32*
___ Green onions *#15, #29*
___ Garlic *#32, #35, #36, #37, #38*
___ Sprouts *#24*

GRAINS/PASTA/RICE

Make sure breads are fat-free.
___ Whole wheat bread
___ French bread
___ Cereal (100% bran, ⅓ cup equals 70 calories and no more than 1.4 grams fat)
___ Cereal (with less than 1 gram fat per serving)
___ Brown rice *#34, #36*

___ Rigatoni or ziti *#37*
___ Rolled oats *#31*
___ Bagels
___ Noodles *#32*
___ English muffins
___ Dinner rolls
___ Pita pockets *#24*
___ Wheat bran *#33*

DAIRY/EGGS

___ Skim milk *#7, #12, #15, #29, #50*
___ Yoplait fat-free light yogurt
___ Fat-free cream cheese
___ Fat-free ricotta cheese *#32*
___ Buttermilk *#12, #33, #51*
___ Eggs or egg substitute *#7, #12, #31, #33, #50, #51*

___ Margarine *#19, #30*
___ Light margarine *#33*
___ Fat-free sour cream *#28*
___ Fat-free plain yogurt *#29, #30*
___ Parmesan cheese *#32, #37*
___ Low-fat cheddar cheese *#15*
___ Fat-free cheese slices *#19, #24*
___ Powdered milk *#31*

Note: Items to be used in recipes are followed by the recipe numbers from Resource 1.

MEAT/POULTRY/FISH

___ Chicken breasts *#35*

___ Cod or other whitefish *#50*

___ Salmon, fresh *#52*

JUICE/SNACKS/DESSERTS

___ Orange juice *#51*

___ Orville Redenbacher Smart-
Pop popcorn

___ Snyder's sourdough pretzels

___ Betty Crocker low-fat brownie
mix

___ Healthy Choice low-fat ice cream

___ Mr. Phipps pretzels

___ Low-calorie cranberry juice

___ Apple juice

___ Fat-free hot fudge sauce

___ Apple pie, fresh or frozen

STAPLES

___ Ketchup *#35*

___ Cornstarch *#37*

___ Molasses *#31*

___ Honey *#7, #12, #33, #35, #51*

___ Fruit spread (no sugar added)

___ Fat-free salad dressing *#8*

___ Brown sugar *#27, #31*

___ Light mayonnaise *#28*

___ Pancake syrup

___ Granulated sugar *#30, #51*

___ Confectioner's sugar *#30*

___ Sweet pickle relish *#8, #28*

___ Worcestershire sauce *#27*

___ Dijon mustard *#8, #27, #35*

___ Vanilla *#7, #12, #51*

___ Olive oil *#36*

___ All-purpose flour *#12, #15,
#23, #30, #31, #33, #51*

___ Oat bran *#12*

___ Whole wheat flour *#12, #33*

___ Baking soda *#12, #30, #31,
#33, #51*

___ Baking powder *#12, #30, #31,
#51*

___ Wheat germ *#12*

___ Red wine vinegar *#35*

___ Dry white wine *#52*

SPICES

___ Dry mustard *#50*

___ Marjoram *#23*

___ Chives

___ Salt

___ Cinnamon *#30, #31*

___ Pepper

___ Basil *#32, #37*

___ Oregano *#37, #38*

___ Dill *#28, #36, #52*

___ Parsley *#23, #32, #37, #38*

___ Paprika *#15*

___ Thyme *#23*

___ Ginger *#35*

___ Nutmeg *#31*

___ Chili powder *#38*

___ Cayenne *#35*

MISCELLANEOUS

___ Water-packed tuna, canned *#8*

___ Quick-cooking tapioca *#7*

___ Baked beans, canned *#27*

___ Barbecue sauce *#27, #35*

___ Black-eyed peas, canned *#34*

___ Tomatoes diced with chili seasoning, canned *#34*

___ Kidney beans, canned *#38*

___ Stewed tomatoes, canned *#37*

___ Cut green beans, canned *#37*

___ Fat-free soda crackers *#50*

___ Graham crackers

___ Unsweetened applesauce *#11, #13, #32, #51*

___ Oyster crackers

Target 1700 Menu for Day 15 (Week 3)

	TOTAL FAT (GRAMS)	SATURATED FAT (GRAMS)	CALORIES
Breakfast			
Cold cereal (½ cup)	1.0	0.1	100
Skim milk (½ cup)	0.2	0.1	43
Orange juice (1)	0.4	0.0	110
Bran cereal (⅓ cup)	1.4	0.3	70
Snack			
Apple (1)	0.2	0.1	81
Lunch			
Baked beans (½ cup) *#27*	1.5	0.3	208
Potato salad (½ cup) *#28*	3.5	0.5	166
Tomato (3 slices)	0.0	0.0	12
Snack			
Bagel (1)	1.0	0.1	200
Low-calorie cranberry juice (1 cup)	0.0	0.0	47
Dinner			
Oven crispy fish (1 serving) *#50*	1.7	0.5	166
Easy mashed potatoes (1 cup) *#29*	0.2	0.1	169
Carrots, cooked (½ cup)	0.1	0.0	24
Green beans (½ cup)	0.2	0.0	22
Whole wheat bread (1 slice)	1.0	0.2	65
Apple bread (1 slice) *#51*	0.8	0.2	193
Snack			
Mr. Phipps pretzels (12)	0.0	0.0	75

Note: Recipe numbers follow dishes that appear in Resource 1.

Total fat: 13.2 grams (7%)   *Saturated fat: 2.5 grams*   *Calories: 1751*

Target 1700 Menu for Day 16 (Week 3)

	TOTAL FAT (GRAMS)	SATURATED FAT (GRAMS)	CALORIES
Breakfast			
Cinnamon-raisin biscuit (1) *#30*	4.0	0.7	166
Banana (1)	0.6	0.2	105
Skim milk (1 cup)	0.4	0.3	86
Snack			
Grapefruit (½)	0.1	0.0	38
Lunch			
Grilled cheese (1) *#19*	8.0	1.6	260
Tomato (3 slices)	0.1	0.0	12
Carrot-oatmeal cookies (2) *#31*	0.9	0.1	110
Snack			
Graham crackers (2 squares)	2.6	0.6	108
Fruit spread (2 tablespoons)	0.0	0.0	84
Dinner			
Cheese and noodles (1 serving) *#32*	3.3	1.5	301
Carrots, cooked (½ cup)	0.1	0.0	24
Tapioca pudding (1 cup) *#7*	0.4	0.3	183
Snack			
Cold cereal (½ cup)	1.0	0.1	100
Skim milk (1 cup)	0.8	0.6	86

Note: Recipe numbers follow dishes that appear in Resource 1.

Total fat: 22.3 grams (12%)   Saturated fat: 6.0 grams   Calories: 1663

Target 1700 Menu for Day 17 (Week 3)

	TOTAL FAT (GRAMS)	SATURATED FAT (GRAMS)	CALORIES
Breakfast			
Cold cereal (½ cup)	1.0	0.1	100
Bran cereal (⅓ cup)	1.4	0.3	70
Skim milk (1 cup)	0.4	0.3	86
Strawberries (½ cup)	0.3	0.0	23
Snack			
English muffin (1)	1.0	0.3	140
Fruit spread (2 tablespoons)	0.0	0.0	84
Lunch			
Taco Bell lite soft taco supreme (1)	5.0	2.0	199
Taco Bell cinnamon twists (1 order)	6.0	3.0	139
Snack			
Apple (1)	0.5	0.1	81
Wheat bran muffin (1) *#33*	2.1	0.5	177
Dinner			
Brown rice with black-eyed peas (1 cup) *#34*	1.9	0.2	222
Cauliflower (½ cup)	0.1	0.0	15
Low-fat cheese sauce (1 serving) *#15*	2.4	1.4	121
Carrots, raw (½ cup)	0.1	0.0	24
Whole wheat bread (1 slices)	1.0	0.2	65
Snack			
Yoplait fat-free light yogurt (6 ounces)	0.0	0.0	90
Graham crackers (2 squares)	2.6	0.6	108

Note: Recipe numbers follow dishes that appear in Resource 1.

Total fat: 25.8 grams (13%)   *Saturated fat: 9.0 grams*   *Calories: 1744*

Target 1700 Menu for Day 18 (Week 3)

	TOTAL FAT (GRAMS)	SATURATED FAT (GRAMS)	CALORIES
Breakfast			
Multi-grain pancake (1) *#12*	4.0	0.8	162
Pancake syrup (2 tablespoons)	0.0	0.0	100
Blueberries (½ cup)	0.3	0.0	41
Skim milk (1 cup)	0.4	0.3	86
Snack			
Nectarine (1)	0.6	0.1	67
Lunch			
Potato, baked (1 medium)	0.2	0.1	220
Chives (to taste)	0.0	0.0	0
Fat-free sour cream (4 tablespoons)	0.0	0.0	60
Carrots, raw (½ cup)	0.1	0.0	24
Apple (1)	0.5	0.1	81
Snack			
Wheat bran muffin (1) *#33*	2.1	0.5	177
Orange juice (1 cup)	0.1	0.0	110
Dinner			
Spicy barbecue chicken (1 serving) *#35*	3.6	1.0	178
Green beans and rice (1 serving) *#36*	2.9	0.5	157
Corn on the cob (1 ear)	1.1	0.2	77
Dinner roll (1)	2.0	0.5	85
Snack			
Snyder's sourdough pretzel (1)	0.0	0.0	111

Note: Recipe numbers follow dishes that appear in Resource 1.

Total fat: 17.9 grams (9%)   *Saturated fat: 4.1 grams*   *Calories: 1736*

Target 1700 Menu for Day 19 (Week 3)

	TOTAL FAT (GRAMS)	SATURATED FAT (GRAMS)	CALORIES
Breakfast			
Cold cereal (½ cup)	1.0	0.1	100
Bran cereal (⅓ cup)	1.4	0.3	70
Blueberries (½ cup)	0.3	0.0	41
Skim milk (1 cup)	0.4	0.3	86
Snack			
Bagel (1)	1.5	0.2	185
Fat-free cream cheese (1 ounce)	0.0	0.0	25
Apple juice (½ cup)	0.1	0.0	58
Lunch			
Arby's roast beef deluxe (1)	10.0	3.5	294
Arby's regular french fries (1 order)	13.2	3.0	246
Snack			
Apple (1)	0.2	0.1	81
Dinner			
Salmon with zucchini and mushrooms (1 serving) #52	8.6	1.6	228
French bread (2 slices)	2.0	0.4	140
Betty Crocker low-fat brownie (1)	2.5	0.5	130
Snack			
Yoplait fat-free light yogurt (6 ounces)	0.0	0.0	90

Note: Recipe numbers follow dishes that appear in Resource 1.

Total fat: 41.2 grams (21%)   Saturated fat: 10.0 grams   Calories: 1774

Target 1700 Menu for Day 20 (Week 3)

	TOTAL FAT (GRAMS)	SATURATED FAT (GRAMS)	CALORIES
Breakfast			
Wheat bran muffin (1) *#33*	2.1	0.5	177
Banana (1)	0.6	0.2	105
Skim milk (1 cup)	0.4	0.3	86
Snack			
Bagel (1)	1.5	0.2	185
Fat-free cream cheese (1 ounce)	0.0	0.0	25
Lunch			
Potato soup (1 cup) *#23*	0.4	0.2	133
Pita with veggies (1) *#24*	2.2	0.1	209
Snack			
Pear (1)	0.7	0.0	98
Dinner			
Pasta primavera (1 serving) *#37*	3.9	1.6	336
French bread (1 slice)	1.0	0.1	70
Healthy Choice low-fat ice cream (½ cup)	2.0	1.5	120
Fat-free hot fudge sauce (2 tablespoons)	1.0	0.0	90
Snack			
Yoplait fat-free light yogurt (6 ounces)	0.0	0.0	90

Note: Recipe numbers follow dishes that appear in Resource 1.

Total fat: 15.8 grams (8%)   Saturated fat: 4.7 grams   Calories: 1724

Target 1700 Menu for Day 21 (Week 3)

	TOTAL FAT (GRAMS)	SATURATED FAT (GRAMS)	CALORIES
Breakfast			
Cold cereal (½ cup)	1.0	0.1	100
Bran cereal (⅓ cup)	1.4	0.3	70
Skim milk (1 cup)	0.4	0.3	86
Orange (1)	0.2	0.0	62
Snack			
Yoplait fat-free light yogurt (6 ounces)	0.0	0.0	90
Lunch			
Tuna sandwich:			
Tuna salad (½ cup) *#8*	2.7	0.6	171
Whole wheat bread (2 slices)	2.0	0.4	130
Broccoli, raw (½ cup)	0.2	0.0	12
Carrots, raw (½ cup)	0.1	0.0	35
Snack			
English muffin (1)	1.0	0.3	140
Skim milk (1 cup)	0.4	0.3	86
Dinner			
Veggie chili (1 cup) *#38*	1.1	0.2	193
Oyster crackers (16)	2.0	0.6	76
Apple pie (⅛ of 9" pie)	13.0	5.0	302
Healthy Choice low-fat ice cream (½ cup)	2.0	2.0	120
Snack			
Orville Redenbacher Smart-Pop popcorn (3 cups)	1.0	1.0	50

Note: Recipe numbers follow dishes that appear in Resource 1.

Total fat: 28.5 grams (15%)　　*Saturated fat: 11.1 grams*　*Calories: 1723*

Target 1700 Grocery List—Week 4

PRODUCE

___ Oranges

___ Apples

___ Blueberries, fresh or frozen #33 (if desired)

___ Bananas

___ Strawberries, fresh or frozen #12

___ Grapefruit

___ Grapes

___ Seedless raisins #33 (if desired), #46

___ Cantaloupe

___ Broccoli #39, #48

___ Mushrooms #41

___ Celery #44

___ Carrots #41, #46, #48

___ Cauliflower #39, #48

___ Zucchini #24

___ Potatoes #41

___ Onions #24, #41, #45

___ Tomatoes #24

___ Lima beans

___ Peas #44

___ Sprouts #24

___ Green pepper #24, #44

___ Garlic #32

___ Leeks #41

GRAINS/PASTA/RICE

Make sure breads are fat-free.

___ Whole wheat bread #43

___ French bread

___ Cereal (100% bran, ⅓ cup equals 70 calories and no more than 1.4 grams fat)

___ Cereal (with less than 1 gram fat per serving)

___ Brown rice #45

___ Linguine #39

___ Bagels

___ Pasta shells or spirals #44

___ Pita pockets #24

___ Whole wheat rolls

___ Tortillas #49

___ Barley #41

DAIRY/EGGS

___ Skim milk #12, #39, #42

___ Yoplait fat-free light yogurt

___ Fat-free cottage cheese

___ Fat-free cream cheese

___ Healthy Choice egg substitute (for scrambled eggs)

___ Fat-free ricotta cheese #40

___ Buttermilk #12, #33, #47

___ Eggs or egg substitute #12, #33, #40, #42, #46, #51

___ Lite margarine #33

___ Fat-free sour cream #40

___ Fat-free plain yogurt #44, #46

___ Parmesan cheese #39

___ Low-fat cheddar cheese #45

___ Fat-free cheese slices #24

Note: Items to be used in recipes are followed by the recipe numbers from Resource 1.

MEAT/POULTRY/FISH

___ Chicken breasts *#47*

___ Salmon, fresh

___ Lean rump roast

JUICE/SNACKS/DESSERTS

___ Orange juice

___ Orville Redenbacher Smart-
Pop popcorn

___ Snyder's sourdough pretzels

___ Betty Crocker low-fat brownie mix

___ Healthy Choice low-fat ice
cream

___ Mr. Phipps barbecue tater crisps

___ Tortilla chips

STAPLES

___ Pancake syrup

___ Lemon juice *#44*

___ Cornstarch *#40*

___ Honey *#12, #33, #40, #44, #48*

___ Fruit spread (no sugar added)
#43

___ Granulated sugar *#42, #46*

___ Baking powder *#12, #42*

___ Dijon mustard *#24, #48*

___ Baking soda *#33, #46*

___ Oat bran *#12*

___ Wheat bran *#33*

___ Whole wheat flour *#12, #33,
#46*

___ All-purpose flour *#33, #39,
#42, #46*

___ Wheat germ *#12*

SPICES/FLAVORINGS

___ Oregano *#45*

___ Garlic powder *#45*

___ Basil *#45*

___ Dill *#44, #48*

___ Thyme *#45*

___ Celery seed *#44*

___ Cinnamon *#46*

___ Bay leaf *#41*

___ Nutmeg *#46*

___ Paprika *#44*

___ Cloves *#46*

___ Flavoring (to be used in cheesecake) *#40*

___ Vanilla *#12, #42*

___ Almond extract *#42*

MISCELLANEOUS

___ Water-packed tuna, canned *#44*

___ Fat-free soda crackers

___ Instant chicken bouillon or
bouillon cubes *#39, #41*

___ Fat-free chicken broth *#45*

___ Pine nuts *#39*

___ Peanut butter *#43*

___ Graham cracker crumbs *#40*

___ Lentils *#45*

___ Vegetarian refried beans,
canned *#49*

___ Salsa *#49*

___ Applesauce (unsweetened) *#12,
#42, #46*

Target 1700 Menu for Day 22 (Week 4)

	TOTAL FAT (GRAMS)	SATURATED FAT (GRAMS)	CALORIES
Breakfast			
Cold cereal (½ cup)	1.0	0.1	100
Bran cereal (⅓ cup)	1.4	0.3	70
Skim milk (1 cup)	0.4	0.3	86
Orange (1)	0.2	0.0	62
Snack			
Wheat bran muffin (1) #33	2.1	0.5	177
Lunch			
Pizza Hut Veggie Lover's pan pizza (1 medium slice)	15.0	5.1	249
Snack			
Carrots, raw (½ cup)	0.1	0.0	24
Celery, raw (1 spear)	0.1	0.0	6
Dinner			
Linguine with vegetables (1 serving) #39	6.4	2.4	285
French bread (2 slices)	2.0	0.4	70
Low-fat cheesecake (1 serving) #40	3.1	0.7	268
Snack			
Snyder's sourdough pretzels (2)	0.0	0.0	222

Note: Recipe numbers follow dishes that appear in Resource 1.

Total fat: 31.8 grams (18%)   Saturated fat: 9.8 grams   Calories: 1619

Target 1700 Menu for Day 23 (Week 4)

	TOTAL FAT (GRAMS)	SATURATED FAT (GRAMS)	CALORIES
Breakfast			
Multi-grain pancakes (2) #12	8.0	1.6	324
Pancake syrup (2 tablespoons)	0.0	0.0	100
Skim milk (1 cup)	0.4	0.3	86
Snack			
Yoplait fat-free light yogurt (6 ounces)	0.0	0.0	90
Wheat bran (2 tablespoons, mix with yogurt)	2.0	0.0	40
Lunch			
Mushroom-barley soup (1 cup) #41	0.4	0.1	85
Fat-free soda crackers (4 squares)	1.5	0.5	49
Snack			
Orville Redenbacher Smart-Pop popcorn (3 cups)	1.0	1.0	50
Dinner			
Salmon, broiled (6 ounces)	12.8	1.2	314
Lima beans (½ cup)	0.3	0.1	100
Brown rice (½ cup)	0.9	0.2	109
Pound cake (1 serving) #42	0.3	0.1	235
Strawberries (½ cup)	0.3	0.0	86
Snack			
Snyder's sourdough pretzel (1)	0.0	0.0	111

Note: Recipe numbers follow dishes that appear in Resource 1.

Total fat: 28.9 grams (15%)   Saturated fat: 6.1 grams   Calories: 1779

Target 1700 Menu for Day 24 (Week 4)

	TOTAL FAT (GRAMS)	SATURATED FAT (GRAMS)	CALORIES
Breakfast			
Cold cereal (½ cup)	1.0	0.1	100
Bran cereal (⅓ cup)	1.4	0.3	70
Cantaloupe (½)	0.7	0.1	94
Skim milk (½ cup)	0.2	0.1	43
Snack			
Yoplait fat-free light yogurt (6 ounces)	0.0	0.0	90
Lunch			
Peanut butter sandwich (1) *#43*	18.4	3.2	386
Skim milk (1 cup)	0.4	0.3	86
Snack			
Apple (1)	0.2	0.1	81
Dinner			
Pasta salad with tuna (1 serving) *#44*	1.7	0.4	210
Tomato (2 slices)	0.3	0.0	24
French bread (2 slices)	1.0	0.2	140
Betty Crocker low-fat brownie (1)	2.5	0.5	130
Snack			
Healthy Choice low-fat ice cream (1 cup)	4.0	2.0	240

Note: Recipe numbers follow dishes that appear in Resource 1.

Total fat: 31.8 grams (17%)   Saturated fat: 7.3 grams   Calories: 1694

Target 1700 Menu for Day 25 (Week 4)

	TOTAL FAT (GRAMS)	SATURATED FAT (GRAMS)	CALORIES
Breakfast			
Oats, cooked (1 cup)	2.0	0.2	144
Maple syrup (2 tablespoons)	0.0	0.0	100
Seedless raisins (¼ cup)	0.2	0.0	108
Skim milk (1 cup)	0.4	0.3	86
Orange juice (½ cup)	0.2	0.0	56
Snack			
Yoplait fat-free light yogurt (6 ounces)	0.0	0.0	90
Lunch			
Wendy's grilled chicken sandwich (1)	7.0	1.5	290
Wendy's side salad (1)	3.0	0.0	60
Reduced calorie Italian dressing	3.0	0.0	40
Snack			
Apple (1)	0.2	0.1	81
Dinner			
Lentil casserole (1 serving) *#45*	2.4	1.0	141
Broccoli, cooked (1 cup)	0.4	0.1	46
Tomato (3 slices)	0.1	0.0	12
Low-fat cheesecake (1 serving) *#40*	3.1	0.7	268
Snack			
Healthy Choice low-fat ice cream (½ cup)	2.0	1.5	120

Note: Recipe numbers follow dishes that appear in Resource 1.

Total fat: 24.0 grams (13%)   *Saturated fat: 5.4 grams*   *Calories: 1642*

Target 1700 Menu for Day 26 (Week 4)

	TOTAL FAT (GRAMS)	SATURATED FAT (GRAMS)	CALORIES
Breakfast			
Healthy Choice egg substitute, scrambled (½ cup)	0.0	0.0	50
Whole wheat toast (1 slice)	1.0	0.7	65
Fruit spread (1 tablespoon)	0.0	0.0	42
Grapefruit (½)	0.1	0.0	38
Skim milk (1 cup)	0.4	0.3	86
Snack			
Yoplait fat-free light yogurt (6 ounces)	0.0	0.0	90
Bran cereal (⅓ cup, add to yogurt)	1.4	0.3	70
Lunch			
Potato, baked (1 medium)	0.2	0.1	220
Broccoli, cooked, used as potato topping (½ cup)	0.2	0.0	23
Fat-free cottage cheese (½ cup), may be used as potato topping	0.0	0.0	90
Snack			
Grapes (20)	0.2	0.0	72
Dinner			
Lean rump roast (6 ounces)	5.5	1.9	324
Potato, cooked with roast (½ medium)	0.1	0.0	110
Carrots, cooked with roast (½ cup)	0.1	0.0	35
Peas (½ cup)	0.2	0.0	34
Whole wheat roll (1)	1.7	0.4	52
Carrot cake (1 serving) #46	0.8	0.2	262
Snack			
Orville Redenbacher Smart-Pop popcorn (3 cups)	1.0	1.0	50

Note: Recipe numbers follow dishes that appear in Resource 1.

Total fat: 13.9 grams (7%)   Saturated fat: 4.9 grams   Calories: 1713

Target 1700 Menu for Day 27
(Week 4)

	TOTAL FAT (GRAMS)	SATURATED FAT (GRAMS)	CALORIES
Breakfast			
Cold cereal (½ cup)	1.0	0.1	100
Bran cereal (⅓ cup)	1.4	0.3	70
Strawberries (½ cup)	0.3	0.0	22
Skim milk (1 cup)	0.4	0.3	86
Snack			
Yoplait fat-free light yogurt (6 ounces)	0.0	0.0	90
Lunch			
Pita with veggies (1) *#24*	2.2	0.1	209
Betty Crocker low-fat brownie (1)	2.5	0.5	130
Skim milk (1 cup)	0.4	0.3	86
Snack			
Bagel (1)	1.5	0.2	185
Fat-free cream cheese (2 ounces)	0.0	0.0	50
Dinner			
Buttermilk chicken (1 serving) *#47*	3.5	1.2	175
Mixed vegetables (1 serving) *#48*	0.4	0.0	51
Carrot cake (1 serving) *#46*	0.8	0.2	262
Skim milk (1 cup)	0.4	0.3	86
Snack			
Mr. Phipps barbecue tater crisps (18)	4.0	0.5	130

Note: Recipe numbers follow dishes that appear in Resource 1.

Total fat: 18.4 grams (10%)   *Saturated fat: 4.0 grams*   *Calories: 1732*

Target 1700 Menu for Day 28 (Week 4)

	TOTAL FAT (GRAMS)	SATURATED FAT (GRAMS)	CALORIES
Breakfast			
Cold cereal (½ cup)	1.0	0.1	100
Bran cereal (⅓ cup)	1.4	0.3	70
Skim milk (1 cup)	0.4	0.3	86
Snack			
Banana (1)	0.6	0.3	105
Lunch			
McDonald's chunky chicken salad (1)	5.0	1.1	160
Reduced-calorie French dressing (1 packet)	8.0	1.0	160
McDonald's soft serve cone (1)	<1.0	0.0	120
Snack			
Orville Redenbacher Smart-Pop popcorn (3 cups)	1.0	1.0	50
Dinner			
Vegetarian bean burritos (2) #49	6.4	0.8	290
Brown rice (½ cup)	0.9	0.2	109
Carrots, raw (2 medium)	0.3	0.0	62
Zucchini, raw or cooked (½ cup)	0.1	1.1	14
Tortilla chips (about 11 chips)	7.0	0.5	150
Salsa (¼ cup)	0.0	0.0	20
Snack			
Healthy Choice low-fat ice cream (½ cup)	2.0	1.5	120

Note: Recipe numbers follow dishes that appear in Resource 1.

Total fat: 35.1 grams (20%)   Saturated fat: 8.2 grams   Calories: 1616

Target 1700
Warthog Alternative *#1*

	TOTAL FAT (GRAMS)	SATURATED FAT (GRAMS)	CALORIES
Breakfast			
Cold cereal (½ cup)	1.0	0.1	100
Banana (1)	0.6	0.1	105
Skim milk (1 cup)	0.4	0.3	86
Snack			
Yoplait fat-free light yogurt (6 ounces)	0.0	0.0	90
Lunch			
Turkey sandwich:			
Turkey (w/o skin, 4 ounces)	2.7	0.8	133
Whole wheat bread (2 slices)	2.0	0.4	130
Lettuce (1 piece)	0.0	0.0	2
Tomato (2 slices)	0.1	0.0	8
Carrots, raw (2 medium)	0.3	0.0	62
Snack			
Oat bran muffin (1) *#1*	1.8	0.3	179
Warthog Dinner			
McDonald's Big Mac (1)	26.0	8.0	510
McDonald's small french fries (1 order)	10.0	2.3	210
McDonald's low-fat hot fudge sundae (1)	5.0	2.4	290
Snack			
Orville Redenbacher Smart-Pop popcorn (6 cups)	2.0	2.0	100

Note: Recipe numbers follow dishes that appear in Resource 1.

Total fat: 51.9 grams (23%)   Saturated fat: 16.7 grams   Calories: 2005

Target 1700
Warthog Alternative #2

	TOTAL FAT (GRAMS)	SATURATED FAT (GRAMS)	CALORIES
Breakfast			
Cold cereal (½ cup)	1.0	0.1	100
Banana (1)	0.6	0.1	105
Skim milk (1 cup)	0.4	0.3	86
Snack			
Yoplait fat-free light yogurt (6 ounces)	0.0	0.0	90
Lunch			
Turkey sandwich:			
Turkey (w/o skin, 4 ounces)	2.7	0.8	133
Whole wheat bread (2 slices)	2.0	0.4	130
Lettuce (1 piece)	0.0	0.0	2
Tomato (2 slices)	0.1	0.0	8
Carrots, raw (2 medium)	0.3	0.0	62
Snack			
Oat bran muffin (1) *#1*	1.8	0.3	179
Warthog Dinner			
Pizza Hut supreme Thin `n Crispy pizza (4 slices)	56.0	30.0	1048
Snack			
Orville Redenbacher Smart-Pop popcorn (3 cups)	1.0	1.0	50

Note: Recipe numbers follow dishes that appear in Resource 1.

Total fat: 65.9 grams (30%)   Saturated fat: 33.0 grams   Calories: 1993

Target 1700
Warthog Alternative #3

	TOTAL FAT (GRAMS)	SATURATED FAT (GRAMS)	CALORIES
Breakfast			
Cold cereal (½ cup)	1.0	0.1	100
Banana (1)	0.6	0.1	105
Skim milk (1 cup)	0.4	0.3	86
Snack			
Yoplait fat-free light yogurt (6 ounces)	0.0	0.0	90
Lunch			
Turkey sandwich:			
Turkey (w/o skin, 4 ounces)	2.7	0.8	133
Whole wheat bread (2 slices)	2.0	0.4	130
Lettuce (1 piece)	0.0	0.0	2
Tomato (2 slices)	0.1	0.0	8
Carrots, raw (2 medium)	0.3	0.0	62
Snack			
Oat bran muffin (1) *#1*	1.8	0.3	179
Warthog Dinner			
Kentucky Fried Chicken:			
Original Recipe chicken breast, wing and drumstick	35.0	9.0	640
Mashed potatoes with gravy	5.0	n/a	109
Coleslaw	6.0	n/a	114
Biscuit (1)	12.0	3.2	200
Snack			
Orville Redenbacher Smart-Pop popcorn (6 cups)	2.0	2.0	100

Note: Recipe numbers follow dishes that appear in Resource 1.

Total fat: 68.9 grams (30%)   Saturated fat: 18 grams   Calories: 2058

Target 1700
Warthog Alternative #4

	TOTAL FAT (GRAMS)	SATURATED FAT (GRAMS)	CALORIES
Breakfast			
Cold cereal (½ cup)	1.0	0.1	100
Banana (1)	0.6	0.1	105
Skim milk (1 cup)	0.4	0.3	86
Snack			
Yoplait fat-free light yogurt (6 ounces)	0.0	0.0	90
Lunch			
Turkey sandwich:			
Turkey (w/o skin, 4 ounces)	2.7	0.8	133
Whole wheat bread (2 slices)	2.0	0.4	130
Lettuce (1 piece)	0.0	0.0	2
Tomato (2 slices)	0.1	0.0	8
Carrots, raw (2 medium)	0.3	0.0	62
Snack			
Oat bran muffin (1) *#1*	1.8	0.3	179
Warthog Dinner			
Taco Bell bean burritos (2)	24.0	3.4	782
Taco Bell cinnamon twists (1 order)	6.0	2.0	139
Nachos	18.0	6.0	345
Snack			
Orville Redenbacher Smart-Pop popcorn (6 cups)	2.0	2.0	100

Note: Recipe numbers follow dishes that appear in Resource 1.

Total fat: 58.9 grams (23%)   Saturated fat: 15.4 grams   Calories: 2261

Target 1700
Warthog Alternative #5

	TOTAL FAT (GRAMS)	SATURATED FAT (GRAMS)	CALORIES
Breakfast			
Cold cereal (½ cup)	1.0	0.1	100
Skim milk (½ cup)	0.2	0.1	43
Orange juice (1 cup)	0.4	0.0	110
Snack			
Apple (1)	0.2	0.1	81
Lunch			
Baked beans (½ cup) *#27*	1.5	0.3	208
Potato salad (½ cup) *#28*	3.5	0.5	166
Tomato (3 slices)	0.0	0.0	12
Snack			
Bagel (1)	1.0	0.1	200
Low-calorie cranberry juice (1 cup)	0.0	0.0	47
Warthog Dinner			
Pork loin chop, broiled (6 ounces)	42.0	17.4	550
Easy mashed potatoes (1 cup) *#29*	0.2	0.1	169
Carrots, cooked (½ cup)	0.1	0.0	24
Whole wheat bread (2 slices)	2.0	0.4	130
Snack			
Mr. Phipps pretzels (12)	0.0	0.0	75

Note: Recipe numbers follow dishes that appear in Resource 1.

Total fat: 52.1 grams (24%)   Saturated fat: 19.1 grams   Calories: 1915

Target 2400 Grocery List—Week 1

PRODUCE

___ Apples
___ Blueberries, fresh or frozen *#1*
___ Grapes

___ Pears (for Jell-O)
___ Bananas
___ Strawberries, fresh or frozen *#12*

___ Broccoli *#9, #13*
___ Mushrooms *#9, #10, #13*
___ Celery *#8*
___ Carrots *#9, #10, #13*
___ Cauliflower *#9, #10*
___ Zucchini *#13*
___ Romaine lettuce *#5*
___ Head lettuce *#10*
___ Potatoes

___ Onions *#9, #13*
___ Tomatoes *#10*
___ Cucumbers *#5*
___ Corn on the cob
___ Green pepper *#10*
___ Peas
___ Snow peas *#9*
___ Spinach *#4*
___ Garlic *#13*

GRAINS/PASTA/RICE

Make sure breads are fat-free.
___ English muffin
___ Whole wheat bread
___ French bread
___ Bagels
___ Whole wheat rolls
___ Spaghetti
___ Cereal (100% bran, ⅓ cup
    equals 70 calories and no
    more than 1.4 grams fat)

___ Cereal (with less than 1 gram
    fat per serving)
___ Brown rice *#9*
___ Jumbo pasta shells *#4*
___ Rigatoni or ziti *#5*
___ Fettucine *#13*

DAIRY/EGGS

___ Skim milk *#7, #12, #13*
___ Yoplait fat-free light yogurt
___ Buttermilk *#1, #6, #12*
___ Eggs or egg substitute *#1, #7,*
    #12
___ Light ricotta cheese *#4*
___ Fat-free mozzarella cheese *#4*

___ Low-fat cheddar cheese *#10*
___ Margarine
___ Fat-free sour cream
___ Fat-free plain yogurt *#3, #11*
___ Parmesan cheese *#4, #6, #13*
___ Healthy Choice fat-free mozza-
    rella cheese sticks

Note: Items to be used in recipes are followed by the recipe numbers from Resource 1.

MEAT/POULTRY/FISH

____ Lean sirloin steak
____ Chicken breasts *#6, #9*
____ Turkey breast *#10*

____ Cod or other whitefish *#2*
____ Shrimp *#13*

JUICE/SNACKS/DESSERTS

____ Orange juice
____ Orville Redenbacher Smart-
Pop popcorn
____ Snyder's sourdough pretzels
____ Betty Crocker low-fat brownie
mix

____ Healthy Choice low-fat ice
cream
____ Chocolate chip cookies (135
calories each)
____ Sugar-free Jell-O
____ Fat-free Newtons

STAPLES

____ Molasses *#1*
____ Honey *#1, #5, #7, #12*
____ Fat-free salad dressing *#3, #8*
____ Fat-free Italian dressing
____ Maple syrup *#11*
____ Lemon juice *#2, #3, #5*
____ Sweet pickle relish *#3, #8*
____ Low-sodium soy sauce *#9*
____ Dijon mustard *#8*

____ Vanilla *#7, #12*
____ Olive oil *#5*
____ All-purpose flour *#12*
____ Oat bran *#1, #12*
____ Whole wheat flour *#1, #12*
____ Baking soda *#1, #12*
____ Baking powder *#12*
____ Wheat germ *#12*
____ Poppyseeds *#11*

SPICES

____ Tarragon *#3*
____ Cajun seasoning *#13*
____ Basil *#5*

____ Salt
____ Pepper

MISCELLANEOUS

____ Salmon, canned *#5*
____ Water-packed tuna, canned *#8*
____ Quick-cooking tapioca *#7*

____ Pitted black olives *#5*
____ Fat-free spaghetti sauce *#4*
____ Unsweetened applesauce *#12*

Target 2400 Menu for Day 1 (Week 1)

	TOTAL FAT (GRAMS)	SATURATED FAT (GRAMS)	CALORIES
Breakfast			
Cold cereal (¾ cup)	2.0	0.2	150
Bran cereal (⅓ cup)	1.4	0.3	70
Skim milk (1 cup)	0.4	0.3	86
Banana (1)	0.6	0.1	105
Snack			
Yoplait fat-free light yogurt (6 ounces)	0.0	0.0	90
Lunch			
Wendy's grilled chicken sandwich (1)	7.0	1.5	290
Wendy's side salad (1)	3.0	0.0	60
Wendy's small frosty (1)	10.0	5.0	340
Reduced-calorie Italian dressing (2 tablespoons)	3.0	0.0	40
Snack			
Oat bran muffin (1) *#1*	1.8	0.3	179
Dinner			
Broiled codfish (8 ounces) *#2*	2.0	0.4	236
Tartar sauce (2 tablespoons) *#3*	0.1	0.0	28
Potato, baked (1 medium)	0.2	0.1	220
Broccoli, steamed (1 cup)	0.4	0.1	46
French bread (2 slices)	2.0	0.4	140
Margarine (½ tablespoon)	5.7	1.0	50
Betty Crocker low-fat brownie (1)	2.5	0.5	130
Snack			
Snyder's sourdough pretzel (1)	0.0	0.0	111

Note: Recipe numbers follow dishes that appear in Resource 1.

Total fat: 42.1 grams (16%)   Saturated fat: 10.2 grams   Calories: 2371

Target 2400 Menu for Day 2
(Week 1)

	TOTAL FAT (GRAMS)	SATURATED FAT (GRAMS)	CALORIES
Breakfast			
Cold cereal (1 cup)	2.0	0.2	200
Skim milk (1 cup)	0.4	0.3	86
Banana (1)	0.6	0.1	105
Snack			
Yoplait light fruit yogurt (6 ounces)	0.0	0.0	90
English muffin (1)	1.0	0.3	140
Lunch			
Turkey sandwich:			
Turkey (w/o skin, 4 ounces)	2.7	0.8	133
Whole wheat bread (2 slices)	2.0	0.4	130
Lettuce (1 piece)	0.0	0.0	2
Tomato (2 slices)	0.1	0.0	8
Carrots, raw (2 medium)	0.3	0.0	62
Chocolate chip cookie (1)	6.0	1.9	135
Snack			
Oat bran muffins (2) *#1*	3.6	0.6	358
Skim milk (1 cup)	0.4	0.3	86
Dinner			
Large stuffed pasta shells (3) *#4*	4.8	3.0	232
Tossed salad (2 cups)	0.2	0.0	20
Fat-free Italian dressing (3 tablespoons)	0.0	0.0	42
French bread (2 slices)	2.0	0.4	140
Margarine (½ tablespoon)	5.7	1.1	50
Betty Crocker low-fat brownies (2)	5.0	1.0	260
Snack			
Orville Redenbacher Smart-Pop popcorn (6 cups)	2.0	2.0	100

Note: Recipe numbers follow dishes that appear in Resource 1.

Total fat: 38.8 grams (15%)   *Saturated fat: 12.4 grams*   *Calories: 2379*

Target 2400 Menu for Day 3
(Week 1)

	TOTAL FAT (GRAMS)	SATURATED FAT (GRAMS)	CALORIES
Breakfast			
Cold cereal (1 cup)	2.0	0.2	200
Bran cereal (⅓ cup)	1.4	0.3	70
Skim milk (1 cup)	0.4	0.3	86
Banana (1)	0.6	0.1	105
Orange juice (1 cup)	0.1	0.0	110
Snack			
Grapes (20)	0.2	0.0	72
Lunch			
Salmon salad (1 serving) #5	9.7	0.8	310
French bread (2 slices)	2.0	0.4	140
Margarine (½ tablespoon)	5.7	1.0	50
Chocolate chip cookie (1)	6.0	1.9	135
Snack			
Yoplait fat-free light yogurt (6 ounces)	0.0	0.0	90
English muffin (1)	1.0	0.3	140
Dinner			
Parmesan chicken (1 serving) #6	5.7	2.6	199
Brown rice (¾ cup)	1.0	0.0	180
Peas and carrots (½ cup each)	0.3	0.1	69
Whole wheat bread (2 slices)	2.0	0.4	130
Tapioca pudding (1 cup) #7	0.4	0.3	183
Snack			
Sugar-free Jell-O (1 cup, ½ pear)	0.0	0.0	54

Note: Recipe numbers follow dishes that appear in Resource 1.

Total fat: 38.5 grams (15%)   Saturated fat: 8.7 grams   Calories: 2323

Target 2400 Menu for Day 4
(Week 1)

	TOTAL FAT (GRAMS)	SATURATED FAT (GRAMS)	CALORIES
Breakfast			
Cold cereal (½ cup)	1.0	0.1	100
Skim milk (1 cup)	0.4	0.3	86
Banana (1)	0.6	0.1	105
Snack			
Oat bran muffin (1) *#1*	1.8	0.3	179
Lunch			
McDonald's McLean Deluxe (1)	12.0	4.0	340
McDonald's low-fat hot fudge sundae (1)	5.0	2.4	290
Snack			
Apple (1)	0.5	0.1	81
Bagel (1)	1.0	0.1	200
Dinner			
Spaghetti with sauce (no meat):			
Spaghetti, cooked (1½ cups)	1.5	0.2	315
Fat-free spaghetti sauce (½ cup)	0.0	0.8	94
French bread (1 slice)	1.0	0.2	70
Tossed salad (2 cups)	0.4	0.1	41
Fat-free Italian dressing (3 tablespoons)	0.0	0.0	42
Healthy Choice low-fat ice cream (1 cup)	4.0	2.0	240
Snack			
Snyder's sourdough pretzels (2)	0.0	0.0	222

Note: Recipe numbers follow dishes that appear in Resource 1.

Total fat: 29.2 grams (11%)   Saturated fat: 10.7 grams   Calories: 2405

Target 2400 Menu for Day 5 (Week 1)

	TOTAL FAT (GRAMS)	SATURATED FAT (GRAMS)	CALORIES
Breakfast			
McDonald's hotcakes with margarine and syrup (1 order)	14.0	5.6	560
Orange juice (6 ounces)	0.0	0.0	80
Snack			
Grapes (20)	0.2	0.0	30
Oat bran muffin (1) #1	1.8	0.3	179
Lunch			
Tuna sandwich:			
Tuna salad (1 serving) #8	2.7	0.6	171
Whole wheat bread (2 slices)	2.0	0.4	130
Carrots, raw (2 whole)	0.3	0.0	62
Chocolate chip cookie (1)	6.0	1.9	135
Snack			
Banana (1)	0.6	0.1	105
Fat-free Newtons (4)	0.0	0.0	200
Dinner			
Stir-fry vegetables with chicken (1 serving) #9	11.0	2.1	261
Brown rice (1 cup)	2.0	0.0	240
Sugar-free Jell-O (1 cup, ½ pear)	0.0	0.0	54
Snack			
Healthy Choice low-fat ice cream (1 cup)	4.0	2.0	240

Note: Recipe numbers follow dishes that appear in Resource 1.

Total fat: 44.6 grams (16%)   *Saturated fat: 13.0 grams*   *Calories: 2447*

Target 2400 Menu for Day 6 (Week 1)

	TOTAL FAT (GRAMS)	SATURATED FAT (GRAMS)	CALORIES
Breakfast			
Cold cereal (1 cup)	2.0	0.2	200
Banana (1)	0.6	0.1	105
Skim milk (½ cup)	0.2	0.1	43
Orange juice (1 cup)	0.1	0.0	110
Snack			
Oat bran muffin (1) *#1*	1.8	0.3	179
Yoplait fat-free light yogurt (6 ounces)	0.0	0.0	90
Lunch			
Chef salad (2 cups) *#10*	7.0	3.9	156
Poppyseed dressing (¼ cup) *#11*	0.2	0.0	54
Whole wheat roll (1)	3.4	0.8	52
Snack			
Apple (1)	0.5	0.1	81
Healthy Choice fat-free mozzarella cheese sticks (2)	0.0	0.0	90
Dinner			
Lean sirloin steak, broiled (8-ounce serving)	16.0	6.2	478
Potato, baked (1 medium)	0.2	0.1	220
Fat-free sour cream (4 tablespoons)	0.0	0.0	60
Peas (½ cup)	0.2	0.0	34
Corn on the cob (1 ear)	1.1	0.2	77
French bread (1 slice)	1.0	0.2	70
Betty Crocker low-fat brownies (2)	5.0	1.0	260
Snack			
Sugar-free Jell-O (1 cup, ½ pear)	0.0	0.0	54

Note: Recipe numbers follow dishes that appear in Resource 1.

Total fat: 39.3 grams (15%)   Saturated fat: 13.2 grams   Calories: 2413

Target 2400 Menu for Day 7 (Week 1)

	TOTAL FAT (GRAMS)	SATURATED FAT (GRAMS)	CALORIES
Breakfast			
Multi-grain pancakes *#12* (4 medium size)	16.0	3.2	646
Strawberries, sliced (1 cup)	0.6	0.0	45
Orange juice (½ cup)	0.1	0.0	55
Snack			
Yoplait fat-free light yogurt (6 ounces)	0.0	0.0	90
Bagel (1)	1.5	0.2	185
Lunch			
Tuna sandwich:			
Tuna salad (1 serving) *#8*	2.7	0.6	171
Whole wheat bread (2 slices)	2.0	0.4	130
Carrots, raw (2 medium)	0.3	0.0	62
Snack			
Oat bran muffin (1) *#1*	1.8	0.3	179
Healthy Choice fat-free mozzarella cheese sticks (2)	0.0	0.0	90
Dinner			
Shrimp fettucine (1 serving) *#13*	7.1	3.2	425
Spinach (1 cup)	0.5	0.0	42
French bread (2 slices)	2.0	0.4	140
Margarine (½ tablespoons)	5.7	1.0	50
Snack			
Orville Redenbacher Smart-Pop popcorn (6 cups)	2.0	2.0	100

Note: Recipe numbers follow dishes that appear in Resource 1.

Total fat: 42.3 grams (16%)   Saturated fat: 11.3 grams   Calories: 2410

Target 2400 Grocery List—Week 2

PRODUCE

___ Grapefruit
___ Cantaloupe
___ Apples
___ Seedless raisins *#33*

___ Broccoli *#20, #22*
___ Mushrooms *#10, #22, #25*
___ Celery *#14*
___ Carrots *#10*
___ Cauliflower *#10*
___ Zucchini *#18, #24*
___ Summer squash
___ Head lettuce *#10*
___ Potatoes *#18, #21, #23*
___ Onions *#14, #18, #20, #21,*
    #22, #23, #24
___ Tomatoes *#10, #18, #24*

___ Grapes
___ Strawberries
___ Bananas

___ Cucumbers *#17*
___ Corn on the cob
___ Green pepper *#10, #14, #18,*
    #24
___ Green beans
___ Eggplant *#18, #26*
___ Spinach *#22, #25*
___ Garlic *#13, #14, #21, #22, #26*
___ Asparagus
___ Scallions *#17*
___ Sprouts *#24*
___ Green onions *#15*

GRAINS/PASTA/RICE

Make sure breads are fat-free.
___ Whole wheat bread
___ Sourdough bread
___ French bread
___ Oatmeal
___ English muffins
___ Whole wheat lasagna noodles
    #22, #25
___ Bagels

___ Rice cakes
___ Pita pockets *#24*
___ Ziti *#26*
___ Cereal (100% bran, ⅓ cup
    equals 70 calories and no
    more than 1.4 grams fat)
___ Cereal (with less than 1 gram
    fat per serving)
___ Brown rice *#14, #17, #20*

DAIRY/EGGS

___ Skim milk *#7, #12, #15, #23*
___ Yoplait fat-free light yogurt
___ Healthy Choice egg substitute
___ Eggs or egg substitute *#7, #12,*
    #25, #33
___ Fat-free cheese slices *#19, #24*
___ Fat-free mozzarella cheese *#22*
___ Low-fat cheddar cheese *#10, #15*
___ Parmesan cheese *#20, #22, #26*

___ Fat-free cottage cheese *#20,*
    #25, #26
___ Margarine
___ Lite margarine *#33*
___ Fat-free sour cream
___ Fat-free plain yogurt *#11*
___ Healthy Choice fat-free mozza-
    rella cheese sticks
___ Buttermilk *#12, #33*

MEAT/POULTRY/FISH

___ Chicken breasts #16, #21   ___ Turkey breast #10

JUICE/SNACKS/DESSERTS

___ Orange juice
___ Grape juice
___ Orville Redenbacher Smart-
Pop popcorn
___ Snyder's sourdough pretzels
___ Betty Crocker low-fat brownie
mix
___ Fat-free Newtons

___ Healthy Choice low-fat ice
cream
___ Chocolate syrup
___ Fat-free hot fudge sauce
___ Sugar-free chocolate pudding
___ Chocolate chip cookies (135
calories each)

STAPLES

___ Honey #7, #12, #16, #33
___ Maple syrup #11
___ Poppyseeds #11
___ Lemon juice #16, #17
___ Dijon mustard #16, #24
___ Vanilla #7, #12
___ Olive oil #17, #18
___ All-purpose flour #12, #15,
#23, #33

___ Vinegar #17, #18
___ Wheat germ #12
___ Wheat bran #33
___ Oat bran #12
___ Baking powder #12
___ Whole wheat flour #12, #33
___ Fruit spread (no sugar added)
___ Baking soda #12, #33

SPICES

___ Paprika #15
___ Marjoram #23
___ Oregano #14, #17, #21, #26
___ Parsley #18, #22, #23, #26
___ Cumin #21
___ Cayenne pepper #14

___ Thyme #23
___ Chives #15
___ Basil #18, #26
___ Chili powder #21
___ Salt
___ Pepper

MISCELLANEOUS

___ Red beans, canned #14
___ Green chilies, canned #21
___ Lentils, dry #17
___ Tomatoes, canned #17
___ Garbanzo beans, canned #18
___ Dry white beans #21
___ Quick-cooking tapioca #7

___ Fat-free spaghetti sauce #22,
#25, #26
___ Unsweetened applesauce #12
___ Unsalted pecans
___ Fat-free saltine crackers
___ Peanut butter
___ Corn, canned

Target 2400 Menu for Day 8 (Week 2)

	TOTAL FAT (GRAMS)	SATURATED FAT (GRAMS)	CALORIES
Breakfast			
Oatmeal, cooked (1 cup)	4.0	0.4	145
Orange juice (1 cup)	0.1	0.0	110
Skim milk (1 cup)	0.4	0.3	86
Snack			
Grapes (20)	0.2	0.0	72
Wheat bran muffin (1) *#33*	2.1	0.5	177
Lunch			
Taco Bell lite taco supreme (2)	10.0	4.0	398
Taco Bell seasoned rice (1 order)	3.0	0.0	110
Taco Bell cinnamon twists (1 order)	6.0	3.0	139
Snack			
Orville Redenbacher Smart-Pop popcorn (6 cups)	2.0	2.0	100
Apple (1)	0.5	0.1	81
Dinner			
Red beans and rice (2 servings) *#14*	3.4	0.6	458
Broccoli, cooked (1 cup)	0.4	0.1	46
Low-fat cheese sauce (½ cup) *#15*	2.4	1.4	121
Tomato (3 slices)	0.2	0.0	12
Carrots, cooked (1 cup)	0.2	0.0	70
Snack			
Snyder's sourdough pretzels (2)	0.0	0.0	222

Note: Recipe numbers follow dishes that appear in Resource 1.

Total fat: 34.9 grams (13%)   Saturated fat: 12.4 grams   Calories: 2347

Target 2400 Menu for Day 9 (Week 2)

	TOTAL FAT (GRAMS)	SATURATED FAT (GRAMS)	CALORIES
Breakfast			
English muffin (1)	1.0	0.3	140
Fruit spread (2 tablespoons)	0.0	0.0	84
Cantaloupe (½)	0.7	0.1	94
Skim milk (1 cup)	0.4	0.3	86
Snack			
Yoplait fat-free light yogurt (6 ounces)	0.0	0.0	90
Wheat bran muffin (1) *#33*	2.1	0.5	177
Lunch			
Chef salad (2 cups) *#10*	7.0	3.9	156
Poppyseed dressing (¼ cup) *#11*	0.2	0.0	54
Whole wheat bread (2 slices)	2.0	0.4	130
Chocolate chip cookie (1)	6.0	1.9	135
Snack			
Apple (1)	0.5	0.1	81
Rice cakes (2)	0.0	0.0	70
Dinner			
Chicken with Dijon mustard (2 servings) *#16*	9.8	1.8	410
Lentil salad (1 cup) *#17*	0.6	0.1	65
Asparagus, cooked (1 cup)	0.6	0.2	44
Sugar-free chocolate pudding (1 cup)	1.0	0.0	130
Snack			
Healthy Choice low-fat ice cream (1 cup)	4.0	2.0	240
Chocolate syrup (4 tablespoons)	2.0	0.8	184
Unsalted pecans (½ ounce)	9.0	0.8	93

Note: Recipe numbers follow dishes that appear in Resource 1.

Total fat: 46.9 grams (17%)   Saturated fat: 13.2 grams   Calories: 2463

Target 2400 Menu for Day 10 (Week 2)

	TOTAL FAT (GRAMS)	SATURATED FAT (GRAMS)	CALORIES
Breakfast			
Cold cereal (1 cup)	2.0	0.2	200
Bran cereal (⅓ cup)	1.4	0.3	70
Strawberries (1 cup)	0.6	0.0	45
Skim milk (1 cup)	0.4	0.3	86
Snack			
Yoplait fat-free light yogurt (6 ounces)	0.0	0.0	90
Grape juice (1 cup)	0.2	0.1	155
Wheat bran muffin (1) *#33*	2.1	0.5	177
Lunch			
McDonald's chunky chicken salad (1)	5.0	1.1	160
McDonald's low-fat hot fudge sundae (1)	5.0	2.4	290
Snack			
Apple (1)	0.5	0.1	81
Fat-free Newtons (4)	0.0	0.0	200
Dinner			
Grilled skinless chicken breast (1)	7.6	2.2	193
Vegetable medley (1 serving) *#18*	4.2	0.6	126
French bread (2 slices)	2.0	0.4	140
Margarine (½ tablespoon)	5.7	1.0	50
Snack			
Bagel (1)	1.5	0.2	185
Fruit spread (2 tablespoons)	0.0	0.0	84
Skim milk (1 cup)	0.4	0.3	86

Note: Recipe numbers follow dishes that appear in Resource 1.

Total fat: 38.6 grams (14%)   Saturated fat: 9.7 grams   Calories: 2418

Target 2400 Menu for Day 11 (Week 2)

	TOTAL FAT (GRAMS)	SATURATED FAT (GRAMS)	CALORIES
Breakfast			
Oatmeal, cooked (⅔ cup uncooked oats)	4.0	0.4	200
Banana (1)	0.6	0.1	105
Skim milk (1 cup)	0.4	0.3	86
Snack			
Yoplait fat-free light yogurt (6 ounces)	0.0	0.0	90
English muffin (1)	1.0	0.3	140
Fruit spread (1 tablespoon)	0.0	0.0	42
Lunch			
Grilled cheese #19	8.0	1.6	260
Tomato (2 slices)	0.1	0.0	8
Carrots, raw (½ cup)	0.1	0.0	24
Snack			
Orville Redenbacher Smart-Pop popcorn (6 cups)	2.0	2.0	100
Dinner			
Grilled skinless chicken breast	7.6	2.2	193
Broccoli-rice casserole (2 servings) #20	10.6	5.8	442
Summer squash, cooked (1 cup)	0.6	0.1	36
Whole wheat bread (2 slices)	2.0	0.4	130
Margarine (½ tablespoon)	5.7	1.0	50
Betty Crocker low-fat brownies (2)	2.0	2.0	200
Snack			
Snyder's sourdough pretzels (2)	0.0	0.0	222
Healthy Choice fat-free mozzarella cheese sticks (2)	0.0	0.0	90

Note: Recipe numbers follow dishes that appear in Resource 1.

Total fat: 44.7 grams (17%)   Saturated fat: 16.2 grams   Calories: 2418

Target 2400 Menu for Day 12
(Week 2)

	TOTAL FAT (GRAMS)	SATURATED FAT (GRAMS)	CALORIES
Breakfast			
Healthy Choice egg substitute, scrambled (½ cup)	0.0	0.0	50
Whole wheat bread (2 slices)	2.0	0.4	130
Margarine (½ tablespoons)	5.7	1.1	50
Fruit spread (2 tablespoons)	0.0	0.0	84
Unsweetened applesauce (½ cup)	0.2	0.0	52
Skim milk (1 cup)	0.4	0.3	86
Snack			
Apple (1)	0.5	0.1	81
Wheat bran muffin (1) *#33*	2.1	0.5	177
Lunch			
White bean chili (2 servings) *#21*	5.8	1.4	470
Fat-free saltine crackers (10)	0.0	0.0	100
Snack			
Banana (1)	0.6	0.1	105
Healthy Choice low-fat ice cream (½ cup)	2.0	1.5	120
Chocolate syrup (2 tablespoons)	1.0	0.4	92
Dinner			
Vegetable lasagna (1 serving) *#22*	6.9	3.6	300
Carrots, cooked (1 cup)	0.1	0.0	35
Green beans (1 cup)	0.2	0.0	50
Corn (½ cup)	1.1	0.2	89
French bread (2 slices)	1.0	0.2	140
Sugar-free chocolate pudding (1 cup)	1.0	0.0	130
Snack			
Orville Redenbacher Smart-Pop popcorn (6 cups)	2.0	2.0	100

Note: Recipe numbers follow dishes that appear in Resource 1.

Total fat: 32.6 grams (12%)   Saturated fat: 11.8 grams   Calories: 2441

Target 2400 Menu for Day 13 (Week 2)

	TOTAL FAT (GRAMS)	SATURATED FAT (GRAMS)	CALORIES
Breakfast			
Bagel (1)	1.5	0.2	185
Margarine (½ tablespoon)	5.7	1.0	50
Fruit spread (2 tablespoons)	0.0	0.0	84
Grapefruit (½)	0.1	0.0	38
Snack			
Peanut butter and crackers:			
4 fat-free saltines and 2 tablespoons peanut butter	18.0	3.3	221
Banana (1)	0.6	0.1	105
Lunch			
Potato soup (2 servings) *#23*	0.8	0.4	266
Pita with veggies (1) *#24*	2.2	0.1	209
Snack			
Apple (1)	0.5	0.1	81
Healthy Choice fat-free mozzarella cheese sticks (2)	0.0	0.0	90
Dinner			
Spinach mushroom lasagna (2 servings) *#25*	2.0	0.0	470
Tossed salad (2 cups)	0.2	0.0	41
Poppyseed dressing (1 serving) *#11*	0.2	0.0	54
Sourdough bread (2 slices)	1.0	0.0	136
Snack			
Healthy Choice low-fat ice cream (1 cup)	4.0	2.0	240
Fat-free hot fudge sauce (4 tablespoons)	0.0	0.0	180

Note: Recipe numbers follow dishes that appear in Resource 1.

Total fat: 36.8 grams (13%)   Saturated fat: 7.2 grams   Calories: 2450

Target 2400 Menu for Day 14 (Week 2)

	TOTAL FAT (GRAMS)	SATURATED FAT (GRAMS)	CALORIES
Breakfast			
Cold cereal (1 cup)	1.0	0.2	200
Skim milk (1 cup)	0.4	0.3	86
Seedless raisins (¼ cup)	0.3	0.1	108
Orange juice (1 cup)	0.4	0.0	110
Snack			
Banana (1)	0.6	0.1	105
Lunch			
Potato, baked (1 medium)	0.2	0.1	270
Fat-free sour cream (4 tablespoons)	0.0	0.0	60
Carrots, raw or steamed (½ cup)	0.1	0.0	24
Broccoli, raw or steamed (1 cup)	0.4	0.0	24
Whole wheat bread (1 slice)	1.0	0.2	65
Snack			
Cantaloupe (½)	0.7	0.1	94
Fat-free cottage cheese (½ cup)	0.0	0.0	90
Dinner			
Eggplant Parmesan with pasta (2 servings) #26	13.8	7.4	600
Corn on the cob (1 ear)	1.1	0.2	77
French bread (2 slices)	1.0	0.2	140
Margarine (½ tablespoon)	5.7	1.0	50
Tapioca pudding (1 cup) #7	0.4	0.3	183
Snack			
Orville Redenbacher Smart-Pop popcorn (6 cups)	2.0	2.0	100

Note: Recipe numbers follow dishes that appear in Resource 1.

Total fat: 29.1 grams (11%)   Saturated fat: 12.2 grams   Calories: 2386

Target 2400 Grocery List—Week 3

PRODUCE

___ Oranges
___ Granny Smith apples *#51*
___ Blueberries, fresh or frozen *#33*
___ Bananas
___ Strawberries, fresh or frozen *#12*

___ Grapefruit
___ Pears
___ Seedless raisins *#30, #31, #33, #51*
___ Nectarines

___ Broccoli
___ Mushrooms *#37, #52*
___ Celery *#8, #28*
___ Carrots *#31, #37*
___ Cauliflower
___ Zucchini *#24, #38, #52*
___ Potatoes *#23, #28*
___ Onions *#23, #24, #28, #36, #38*

___ Tomatoes *#24, #38*
___ Lemon *#50*
___ Green beans *#36*
___ Corn on the cob
___ Green pepper *#24, #38*
___ Spinach *#32*
___ Green onions *#29*
___ Garlic *#32, #35, #36, #37, #38*
___ Sprouts *#24*

GRAINS/PASTA/RICE

Make sure breads are fat-free.
___ Whole wheat bread
___ French bread
___ Cereal (100% bran, ⅓ cup equals 70 calories and no more than 1.4 grams fat)
___ Cereal (with less than 1 gram fat per serving)
___ Brown rice *#34, #36*

___ Rigatoni or ziti *#37*
___ Rolled oats *#31*
___ Bagels
___ Noodles *#32*
___ English muffins
___ Dinner rolls
___ Pita pockets *#24*
___ Wheat bran *#33*

DAIRY/EGGS

___ Skim milk *#7, #12, #23, #29, #50*
___ Yoplait fat-free light yogurt
___ Fat-free cottage cheese
___ Fat-free cream cheese
___ Healthy Choice egg substitute *#51*
___ Fat-free ricotta cheese *#32, #40*
___ Buttermilk *#12, #33, #51*

___ Eggs or egg substitute *#7, #12, #33, #40, #50, #51*
___ Margarine *#30, #40*
___ Lite margarine *#33*
___ Fat-free sour cream *#28, #40*
___ Fat-free plain yogurt *#29, #30, #40*
___ Parmesan cheese *#32, #37*
___ Fat-free cheese slices *#19, #24*
___ Powdered milk *#31*

Note: Items to be used in recipes are followed by the recipe numbers from Resource 1.

MEAT/POULTRY/FISH

___ Cod or other whitefish *#50*   ___ Salmon, fresh *#52*
___ Chicken breasts *#35*

JUICE/SNACKS/DESSERTS

___ Orange juice *#51*
___ Orville Redenbacher Smart-
  Pop popcorn
___ Snyder's sourdough pretzels
___ Betty Crocker low-fat brownie
  mix
___ Healthy Choice low-fat ice
  cream

___ Mr. Phipps pretzels
___ Low-calorie cranberry juice
___ Apple juice
___ Fat-free hot fudge sauce
___ Fat-free Newtons
___ Apple pie, fresh or frozen

STAPLES

___ Ketchup *#35*
___ Cornstarch *#37, #40*
___ Molasses *#31*
___ Honey *#7, #12, #33, #35, #40,*
  #51
___ Fruit spread (no sugar added)
___ Fat-free salad dressing *#8*
___ Brown sugar *#27, #31*
___ Light mayonnaise *#28*
___ Pancake syrup
___ Granulated sugar *#30, #51*
___ Confectioner's sugar *#30*
___ Sweet pickle relish *#8, #28*
___ Worcestershire sauce *#27*
___ Dijon mustard *#8, #24, #27,*
  #35

___ Vanilla *#7, #40, #51*
___ Olive oil *#36*
___ All-purpose flour *#12, #23,*
  #30, #31, #33, #51
___ Oat bran *#12*
___ Whole wheat flour *#12, #33*
___ Baking soda *#12, #30, #31,*
  #33, #51
___ Baking powder *#12, #30, #31,*
  #33, #51
___ Wheat germ *#12*
___ Red wine vinegar *#35*
___ Dry white wine *#52*

SPICES

___ Cinnamon *#30, #31*
___ Marjoram *#23*
___ Salt
___ Cayenne pepper *#35*
___ Pepper
___ Basil *#32, #37*
___ Oregano *#37, #38*
___ Chives

___ Dill *#28, #36, #52*
___ Parsley *#23, #32, #37, #38*
___ Nutmeg *#31*
___ Thyme *#23*
___ Ginger *#35*
___ Dry mustard *#50*
___ Chili powder *#38*

MISCELLANEOUS

___ Water-packed tuna, canned *#8*

___ Quick-cooking tapioca *#7*

___ Baked beans, canned *#27*

___ Barbecue sauce *#27, #35*

___ Black-eyed peas, canned *#34*

___ Tomatoes, canned *#34*

___ Kidney beans, canned *#38*

___ Stewed tomatoes, canned *#37*

___ Cut green beans, canned *#37*

___ Fat-free soda crackers *#50*

___ Graham crackers *#40*

___ Unsweetened applesauce *#12, #31, #51*

___ Oyster crackers

Target 2400 Menu for Day 15 (Week 3)

	TOTAL FAT (GRAMS)	SATURATED FAT (GRAMS)	CALORIES
Breakfast			
Cold cereal (1 cup)	2.0	0.2	200
Skim milk (½ cup)	0.2	0.1	43
Orange juice (1)	0.4	0.0	110
Snack			
Apple (1)	0.2	0.1	81
Wheat bran muffin (1) *#33*	2.1	0.5	177
Lunch			
Baked beans (1 cup) *#27*	3.0	0.6	416
Potato salad (½ cup) *#28*	3.5	0.5	166
Tomato (3 slices)	0.0	0.0	12
Snack			
Apple bread (1 slice) *#51*	0.8	0.2	193
Fat-free cream cheese (2 ounces)	0.0	0.0	50
Low-calorie cranberry juice (1 cup)	0.0	0.0	47
Dinner			
Oven crispy fish (2 servings) *#50*	3.4	1.0	332
Easy mashed potatoes (1 cup) *#29*	0.2	1.0	169
Carrots, cooked (½ cup)	0.1	0.0	24
Whole wheat bread (2 slices)	2.0	0.4	130
Healthy Choice low-fat ice cream (1 cup)	4.0	2.0	240
Snack			
Mr. Phipps pretzels (12)	0.0	0.0	75

Note: Recipe numbers follow dishes that appear in Resource 1.

Total fat: 21.9 grams (8%)   *Saturated fat: 5.7 grams*   *Calories: 2465*

Target 2400 Menu for Day 16 (Week 3)

	TOTAL FAT (GRAMS)	SATURATED FAT (GRAMS)	CALORIES
Breakfast			
Cinnamon-raisin biscuits (2) *#30*	8.0	1.4	332
Banana (1)	0.6	0.2	105
Skim milk (1 cup)	0.4	0.3	86
Snack			
Grapefruit (½)	0.1	0.0	38
Lunch			
Grilled cheese *#19*	8.0	1.6	260
Tomato (3 slices)	0.1	0.0	12
Mr. Phipps pretzels (12)	0.0	0.0	75
Carrot-oatmeal cookies (2) *#31*	0.9	0.1	110
Snack			
Graham crackers (4 squares)	5.2	1.2	216
Fruit spread (2 tablespoons)	0.0	0.0	84
Dinner			
Cheese and noodles (2 servings) *#32*	6.6	3.0	602
Carrots, cooked (½ cup)	0.1	0.0	24
Tapioca pudding (1 cup) *#7*	0.4	0.3	183
French bread (2 slices)	2.0	0.4	140
Snack			
Orville Redenbacher Smart-Pop popcorn (6 cups)	2.0	2.0	100

Note: Recipe numbers follow dishes that appear in Resource 1.

Total fat: 34.4 grams (13%)   Saturated fat: 10.5 grams   Calories: 2367

Target 2400 Menu for Day 17
(Week 3)

	TOTAL FAT (GRAMS)	SATURATED FAT (GRAMS)	CALORIES
Breakfast			
Cold cereal (1 cup)	2.0	0.2	200
Bran cereal (⅓ cup)	1.4	0.3	70
Skim milk (1 cup)	0.4	0.3	86
Strawberries (½ cup)	0.3	0.0	23
Snack			
English muffin (1)	1.0	0.3	140
Fruit spread (2 tablespoons)	0.0	0.0	84
Orange juice (1 cup)	0.1	0.0	110
Lunch			
Taco Bell lite soft taco supreme (2)	10.0	4.0	398
Taco Bell cinnamon twists (1 order)	6.0	3.0	139
Snack			
Apple (1)	0.5	0.1	81
Dinner			
Brown rice with black-eyed peas (2 cups) *#34*	3.8	0.4	444
Carrots, raw (½ cup)	0.1	0.0	24
Whole wheat bread (2 slices)	2.0	0.4	130
Margarine (½ tablespoon)	5.7	1.0	50
Low-fat cheesecake (1) *#40*	3.1	0.7	268
Snack			
Yoplait fat-free light yogurt (6 ounces)	0.0	0.0	90

Note: Recipe numbers follow dishes that appear in Resource 1.

Total fat: 36.4 grams (14%)   Saturated fat: 10.7 grams   Calories: 2337

Target 2400 Menu for Day 18
Week 3

	TOTAL FAT (GRAMS)	SATURATED FAT (GRAMS)	CALORIES
Breakfast			
Multi-grain pancakes (2) #12	8.0	1.6	324
Pancake syrup (2 tablespoons)	0.0	0.0	100
Blueberries (1 cup)	0.6	0.0	82
Skim milk (1 cup)	0.4	0.3	86
Margarine (½ tablespoon)	5.7	1.0	50
Snack			
Nectarine (1)	0.6	0.1	67
Yoplait fat-free light yogurt (6 ounces)	0.0	0.0	90
Lunch			
Potato, baked (1 medium)	0.2	0.1	220
Chives (to taste)	0.0	0.0	0
Fat-free sour cream (4 tablespoons)	0.0	0.0	60
Margarine (1 tablespoon)	11.4	2.0	100
Carrots, raw (½ cup)	0.1	0.0	24
Apple (1)	0.5	0.1	81
Snack			
Wheat bran muffin (1) #33	2.1	0.5	177
Orange juice (1 cup)	0.1	0.0	110
Dinner			
Spicy barbecue chicken (2 servings) #35	7.2	2.0	356
Green beans and rice (1 serving) #36	2.9	0.5	157
Corn on the cob (1 ear)	1.1	0.2	77
Dinner roll (2)	4.0	1.0	170
Snack			
Snyder's sourdough pretzel (1)	0.0	0.0	111

Note: Recipe numbers follow dishes that appear in Resource 1.

Total fat: 44.9 grams (17%)   Saturated fat: 9.4 grams   Calories: 2442

Target 2400 Menu for Day 19
Week 3

	TOTAL FAT (GRAMS)	SATURATED FAT (GRAMS)	CALORIES
Breakfast			
Cold cereal (1 cup)	2.0	0.2	200
Bran cereal (⅓ cup)	1.4	0.3	70
Blueberries (½ cup)	0.3	0.0	41
Skim milk (1 cup)	0.4	0.3	86
Snack			
Bagel (1)	1.5	0.2	185
Fat-free cream cheese (1 ounce)	0.0	0.0	25
Apple juice (1 cup)	0.2	0.0	116
Lunch			
Arby's roast beef deluxe (1)	10.0	3.5	294
Arby's regular french fries (1 order)	13.2	3.0	246
Snack			
Apple (1)	0.2	0.1	81
Skim milk (1 cup)	0.4	0.3	86
Dinner			
Salmon with zucchini and mushrooms (1 serving) *#52*	8.6	1.6	228
French bread (2 slices)	2.0	0.4	140
Betty Crocker low-fat brownies (2)	2.0	2.0	200
Healthy Choice low-fat ice cream (1 cup)	4.0	2.0	240
Snack			
Yoplait fat-free light yogurt (6 ounces)	0.0	0.0	90

Note: Recipe numbers follow dishes that appear in Resource 1.

Total fat: 46.2 grams (18%)   Saturated fat: 13.9 grams   Calories: 2328

Target 2400 Menu for Day 20
Week 3

	TOTAL FAT (GRAMS)	SATURATED FAT (GRAMS)	CALORIES
Breakfast			
Wheat bran muffin (1) *#33*	2.1	0.5	177
Banana (1)	0.6	0.2	105
Skim milk (1 cup)	0.4	0.3	86
Snack			
Bagel (1)	1.5	0.2	185
Fat-free cream cheese (2 ounces)	0.0	0.0	50
Lunch			
Potato soup (1 cup) *#23*	0.4	0.2	133
Pita with veggies (1) *#24*	2.2	0.1	209
Snack			
Pear (1)	0.7	0.0	98
Fat-free Newtons (2)	0.0	0.0	100
Dinner			
Pasta primavera (2 servings) *#37*	7.8	3.2	672
French bread (2 slices)	2.0	0.2	140
Healthy Choice low-fat ice cream (1 cup)	4.0	2.0	240
Fat-free hot fudge sauce (4 tablespoons)	1.0	0.0	90
Snack			
Yoplait fat-free light yogurt (6 ounces)	0.0	0.0	90

Note: Recipe numbers follow dishes that appear in Resource 1.

Total fat: 22.7 grams (9%)   *Saturated fat: 6.9 grams*   *Calories: 2375*

Target 2400 Menu for Day 21
Week 3

	TOTAL FAT (GRAMS)	SATURATED FAT (GRAMS)	CALORIES
Breakfast			
Cold cereal (1 cup)	2.0	0.2	200
Bran cereal (⅓ cup)	1.4	0.3	70
Skim milk (1 cup)	0.4	0.3	86
Orange (1)	0.2	0.0	62
Snack			
Yoplait fat-free light yogurt (6 ounces)	0.0	0.0	90
Fat-free Newtons (2)	0.0	0.0	100
Lunch			
Tuna sandwich:			
Tuna salad (½ cup) #8	2.7	0.6	171
Whole wheat bread (2 slices)	2.0	0.4	130
Broccoli, raw (½ cup)	0.2	0.0	12
Carrots, raw (½ cup)	0.1	0.0	35
Fat-free cottage cheese (½ cup)	0.0	0.0	90
Snack			
Banana (1)	0.6	0.1	105
English muffin (1)	1.0	0.3	140
Fruit spread (2 tablespoons)	0.0	0.0	84
Dinner			
Veggie chili (2 cups) #38	2.2	0.4	386
Oyster crackers (16)	2.0	0.6	76
Apple pie (⅛ of 9" pie)	13.0	5.0	302
Healthy Choice low-fat ice cream (½ cup)	2.0	1.0	120
Snack			
Orville Redenbacher Smart-Pop popcorn (6 cups)	2.0	2.0	100

Note: Recipe numbers follow dishes that appear in Resource 1.

Total fat: 31.8 grams (12%)   Saturated fat: 11.2 grams   Calories: 2359

Target 2400 Grocery List—Week 4

PRODUCE

___ Oranges
___ Apples
___ Blueberries, fresh or frozen *#33*
___ Bananas
___ Strawberries, fresh or frozen
      #12, #42

___ Grapefruit
___ Grapes
___ Seedless raisins *#46*

___ Cantaloupe
___ Broccoli *#39, #48*
___ Mushrooms *#41*
___ Celery *#44*
___ Carrots *#41, #46, #48*
___ Cauliflower *#39, #48*
___ Zucchini *#24*
___ Potatoes *#41*
___ Onions *#24, #41, #45*

___ Tomatoes *#24*
___ Lima beans
___ Peas *#44*
___ Brussels sprouts
___ Sprouts *#24*
___ Green pepper *#24, #44*
___ Leeks *#41*
___ Green onion *#44*

GRAINS/PASTA/RICE

Make sure breads are fat-free.
___ Whole wheat bread *#43*
___ French bread
___ Cereal (100% bran, ⅓ cup
      equals 70 calories and no
      more than 1.4 grams fat)
___ Cereal (with less than 1 gram
      fat per serving)
___ Brown rice *#45*

___ Linguine *#39*
___ Bagels
___ Pasta shells or spirals *#44*
___ Pita pockets *#24*
___ Wheat bran *#33*
___ Whole wheat rolls
___ Tortillas *#49*
___ Barley *#41*
___ English muffin

DAIRY

___ Skim milk *#12, #39, #42*
___ Yoplait fat-free light yogurt
___ Fat-free cream cheese
___ Healthy Choice egg substitute
      (for scrambled eggs)
___ Fat-free ricotta cheese *#40*
___ Buttermilk *#12, #33, #47*
___ Eggs or egg substitute *#12,
      #33, #40, #42, #46, #51*

___ Margarine *#40*
___ Light margarine *#33*
___ Fat-free sour cream *#40*
___ Fat-free plain yogurt *#40, #44,
      #46*
___ Parmesan cheese *#39*
___ Low-fat cheddar cheese *#45*
___ Fat-free cheese slices *#24*

Note: Items to be used in recipes are followed by the recipe numbers from Resource 1.

MEAT/POULTRY/FISH

___ Chicken breasts *#47*
___ Salmon, fresh

___ Lean rump roast

JUICE/SNACKS/DESSERTS

___ Orange juice
___ Orville Redenbacher Smart-
    Pop popcorn
___ Snyder's sourdough pretzels
___ Fat-free Newtons
___ Betty Crocker low-fat brownie mix

___ Healthy Choice low-fat ice
    cream
___ Mr. Phipps barbecue tater crisps
___ Tortilla chips

STAPLES

___ Pancake syrup
___ Maple syrup
___ Lemon juice *#44*
___ Cornstarch *#40*
___ Honey *#12, #33, #40, #44, #48*
___ Fruit spread (no sugar added)
    #43
___ Granulated sugar *#42, #46*

___ Dijon mustard *#24, #48*
___ Baking powder *#12, #42*
___ Oat bran *#12*
___ All-purpose flour *#12, #33,
    #39, #42, #46*
___ Whole wheat flour *#12, #33, #46*
___ Wheat germ *#12*
___ Baking soda *#12, #33, #46*

SPICES/FLAVORINGS

___ Oregano *#45*
___ Garlic powder *#45*
___ Basil *#45*
___ Dill *#44, #48*
___ Thyme *#45*
___ Celery seed *#44*
___ Almond extract *#42*

___ Cinnamon *#46*
___ Bay leaf *#41*
___ Nutmeg *#46*
___ Paprika *#44*
___ Cloves *#46*
___ Vanilla or other flavoring for
    cheesecake *#12, #40, #42*

MISCELLANEOUS

___ Water-packed tuna, canned *#44*
___ Fat-free soda crackers
___ Instant chicken bouillon *#39,
    #41, #42, #44, #45*
___ Fat-free chicken broth, canned
    #45
___ Pine nuts *#39*
___ Peanut butter *#43*

___ Graham cracker crumbs *#40*
___ Lentils *#45*
___ Vegetarian refried beans *#49*
___ Salsa *#49*
___ Applesauce (unsweetened) *#12,
    #42, #46*
___ Chocolate syrup

Target 2400 Menu for Day 22 (Week 4)

	TOTAL FAT (GRAMS)	SATURATED FAT (GRAMS)	CALORIES
Breakfast			
Wheat bran muffin (2) *#33*	4.2	1.0	354
Skim milk (1 cup)	0.4	0.3	86
Orange (1)	0.2	0.0	62
Snack			
Yoplait fat-free light yogurt (6 ounces)	0.0	0.0	90
Fat-free Newtons (2)	0.0	0.0	100
Lunch			
Pizza Hut Veggie Lover's pan pizza (2 slices)	30.0	10.2	498
Snack			
Carrots, raw (½ cup)	0.1	0.0	24
Celery, raw (1 spear)	0.1	0.0	6
Bagel (1)	1.0	0.0	200
Fat-free cream cheese (2 ounces)	0.0	0.0	50
Dinner			
Linguine with vegetables (1 serving) *#39*	6.4	2.4	285
French bread (2 slices)	2.0	0.4	70
Margarine (½ tablespoon)	5.7	1.0	50
Low-fat cheesecake (1 serving) *#40*	3.1	0.7	268
Snack			
Snyder's sourdough pretzels (2)	0.0	0.0	222

Note: Recipe numbers follow dishes that appear in Resource 1.

Total fat: 53.2 grams (20%)   Saturated fat: 16.0 grams   Calories: 2365

Target 2400 Menu for Day 23
(Week 4)

	TOTAL FAT (GRAMS)	SATURATED FAT (GRAMS)	CALORIES
Breakfast			
Multi-grain pancakes (2) *#12*	8.0	1.6	324
Pancake syrup (4 tablespoons)	0.0	0.0	200
Skim milk (1 cup)	0.4	0.3	86
Margarine (½ tablespoon)	5.7	1.0	50
Snack			
Yoplait fat-free light yogurt (6 ounce)	0.0	0.0	90
Banana (1)	0.6	0.1	105
Lunch			
Mushroom-barley soup (2 cups) *#41*	0.8	0.2	170
Fat-free soda crackers (4 squares)	1.5	0.5	49
Bean burrito (1) *#49*	3.2	0.4	145
Snack			
Apple (1)	0.5	0.1	81
Dinner			
Salmon, broiled (6 ounces)	12.8	1.2	314
Lima beans (½ cup)	0.3	0.1	100
Brown rice (1 cup)	1.8	0.4	218
Pound cake (1 serving) *#42*	0.3	0.1	235
Strawberries (½ cup)	0.3	0.0	86
Snack			
Snyder's sourdough pretzels (2)	0.0	0.0	222

Note: Recipe numbers follow dishes that appear in Resource 1.

Total fat: 36.2 grams (13%)   *Saturated fat: 6.0 grams*   *Calories: 2475*

Target 2400 Menu for Day 24 (Week 4)

	TOTAL FAT (GRAMS)	SATURATED FAT (GRAMS)	CALORIES
Breakfast			
Cold cereal (1 cup)	2.0	0.2	200
Bran cereal (⅓ cup)	1.4	0.3	70
Cantaloupe (½)	0.7	0.1	94
Skim milk (1 cup)	0.4	0.3	86
Snack			
Yoplait fat-free light yogurt (6 ounces)	0.0	0.0	90
Banana (1)	0.6	0.1	105
Lunch			
Peanut butter sandwich (1) *#43*	18.4	3.2	386
Skim milk (1 cup)	0.4	0.3	86
Carrots, raw (2 medium)	0.3	0.0	62
Snack			
Apple (1)	0.2	0.1	81
English muffin (1)	1.0	0.3	140
Fruit spread (2 tablespoons)	0.0	0.0	84
Dinner			
Pasta salad with tuna (1½ servings) *#44*	2.6	0.6	315
Tomato (2 slices)	0.3	0.0	24
French bread (2 slices)	1.0	0.2	140
Betty Crocker low-fat brownie (1)	2.5	0.5	130
Margarine (½ tablespoon)	5.7	1.1	50
Snack			
Healthy Choice low-fat ice cream (1 cup)	4.0	2.0	240

Note: Recipe numbers follow dishes that appear in Resource 1.

Total fat: 41.5 grams (16%)   Saturated fat: 9.3 grams   Calories: 2383

Target 2400 Menu for Day 25 (Week 4)

	TOTAL FAT (GRAMS)	SATURATED FAT (GRAMS)	CALORIES
Breakfast			
Oats, cooked (1 cup)	2.0	0.2	144
Maple syrup (2 tablespoons)	0.0	0.0	100
Raisins (¼ cup)	0.2	0.0	108
Skim milk (1 cup)	0.4	0.3	86
Orange juice (1 cup)	0.4	0.0	112
Snack			
English muffin (1)	1.0	0.3	140
Fruit spread (2 tablespoons)	0.0	0.0	84
Lunch			
Wendy's grilled chicken sandwich (1)	7.0	0.0	290
Wendy's side salad (1)	3.0	0.0	60
Reduced calorie Italian dressing	3.0	0.0	40
Snack			
Apple (1)	0.2	0.1	81
Fat-free Newtons (4)	0.0	0.0	200
Dinner			
Lentil casserole (2 servings) *#45*	4.8	2.0	282
Broccoli, cooked (1 cup)	0.4	0.1	46
Tomato (3 slices)	0.1	0.0	12
Low-fat cheesecake (1 serving) *#40*	3.1	0.7	268
Snack			
Healthy Choice low-fat ice cream (1 cup)	4.0	3.0	240
Chocolate syrup (2 tablespoons)	1.0	0.4	92

Note: Recipe numbers follow dishes that appear in Resource 1.

Total fat: 30.6 grams (12%)　　*Saturated fat: 7.1 grams*　　*Calories: 2385*

Target 2400 Menu for Day 26 (Week 4)

	TOTAL FAT (GRAMS)	SATURATED FAT (GRAMS)	CALORIES
Breakfast			
Healthy Choice egg substitute, scrambled (1 cup)	0.0	0.0	100
Whole wheat toast (2 slices)	2.0	1.4	130
Fruit spread (2 tablespoons)	0.0	0.0	84
Grapefruit (½)	0.1	0.0	38
Skim milk (1 cup)	0.4	0.3	86
Snack			
Yoplait fat-free light yogurt (6 ounces)	0.0	0.0	90
Lunch			
Wendy's broccoli and cheese potato (1)	14.0	2.5	460
Wendy's small frosty (1)	10.0	5.0	340
Snack			
Grapes (20)	0.2	0.0	72
Fat-free Newtons (2)	0.0	0.0	100
Dinner			
Lean rump roast (6 ounces)	5.5	1.9	324
Potato, cooked with roast (½ medium)	0.1	0.0	110
Carrots, cooked with roast (½ cup)	0.1	0.0	35
Brussels sprouts (½ cup)	0.4	0.1	30
Whole wheat roll (1)	1.7	0.4	52
Carrot cake (1 serving) #46	0.8	0.2	262
Snack			
Orville Redenbacher Smart-Pop popcorn (6 cups)	2.0	2.0	100

Note: Recipe numbers follow dishes that appear in Resource 1.

Total fat: 37.3 grams (14%)   Saturated fat: 13.8 grams   Calories: 2413

Target 2400 Menu for Day 27 (Week 4)

	TOTAL FAT (GRAMS)	SATURATED FAT (GRAMS)	CALORIES
Breakfast			
Cold cereal (1 cup)	2.0	0.2	200
Bran cereal (⅓ cup)	1.4	0.3	70
Strawberries (½ cup)	0.3	0.0	22
Skim milk (1 cup)	0.4	0.3	86
Snack			
Yoplait fat-free light yogurt (6 ounces)	0.0	0.0	90
Wheat bran muffin (1) *#33*	2.1	0.5	177
Lunch			
Pitas with veggies (2) *#24*	4.4	0.2	418
Betty Crocker low-fat brownies (2)	5.0	0.5	260
Skim milk (1 cup)	0.4	0.3	86
Snack			
Bagel (1)	1.5	0.2	185
Fat-free cream cheese (2 ounces)	0.0	0.0	50
Dinner			
Buttermilk chicken (2 servings) *#47*	7.0	2.4	350
Mixed vegetables (1 serving) *#48*	0.4	0.0	51
Carrot cake (1 serving) *#46*	0.8	0.2	262
Snack			
Mr. Phipps barbecue tater crisps (18)	4.0	0.5	130

Note: Recipe numbers follow dishes that appear in Resource 1.

Total fat: 29.7 grams (11%)   Saturated fat: 5.6 grams   Calories: 2437

Target 2400 Menu for Day 28 (Week 4)

	TOTAL FAT (GRAMS)	SATURATED FAT (GRAMS)	CALORIES
Breakfast			
Cold cereal (1 cup)	2.0	0.2	200
Bran cereal (⅓ cup)	1.4	0.3	70
Banana (1)	0.6	0.3	105
Skim milk (1 cup)	0.4	0.3	86
Snack			
Yoplait fat-free light yogurt (6 ounces)	0.0	0.0	90
Lunch			
McDonald's chunky chicken salad (1)	5.0	1.1	160
Reduced-calorie French dressing (1 packet)	8.0	1.0	160
McDonald's low-fat hot fudge sundae (1)	5.0	2.4	290
Snack			
Orville Redenbacher Smart-Pop popcorn (6 cups)	2.0	2.0	100
Dinner			
Vegetarian bean burritos (3) #49	9.6	1.2	435
Brown rice (1 cup)	1.8	0.4	218
Carrots, raw (2 medium)	0.3	0.0	62
Salsa for burritos (½ cup)	0.0	0.0	40
Betty Crocker low-fat brownies (2)	5.0	1.0	260
Snack			
Healthy Choice low-fat ice cream (1 cup)	4.0	2.0	240

Note: Recipe numbers follow dishes that appear in Resource 1.

Total fat: 45.1 grams (16%)   Saturated fat: 12.2 grams   Calories: 2516

Target 2400
Warthog Alternative #1

	TOTAL FAT (GRAMS)	SATURATED FAT (GRAMS)	CALORIES
Breakfast			
Cold cereal (1 cup)	2.0	0.2	200
Banana (1)	0.6	0.1	105
Skim milk (1 cup)	0.4	0.3	86
Whole wheat bread (1 slice)	2.0	0.2	65
Margarine (½ tablespoon)	5.7	1.1	50
Fruit spread (1 tablespoon)	0.0	0.0	42
Snack			
Yoplait fat-free light yogurt (6 ounces)	0.0	0.0	90
Lunch			
Turkey sandwich:			
Turkey (w/o skin, 4 ounces)	2.7	0.8	133
Whole wheat bread (2 slices)	2.0	0.4	130
Lettuce (1 piece)	0.0	0.0	2
Tomato (2 slices)	0.1	0.0	8
Carrots, raw (2 medium)	0.3	0.0	62
Snack			
Apple (1)	0.5	0.1	81
Oat bran muffin (1) *#1*	1.8	0.3	179
Warthog Dinner			
McDonald's Big Mac (1)	26.0	8.0	510
McDonald's large french fries (1 order)	22.0	5.0	450
McDonald's low-fat hot fudge sundae (1)	5.0	2.4	290
Snack			
Orville Redenbacher Smart-Pop popcorn (6 cups)	2.0	2.0	100

Note: Recipe numbers follow dishes that appear in Resource 1.

Total fat: 73.1 grams (26%)   Saturated fat: 20.9 grams   Calories: 2583

Target 2400
Warthog Alternative *#2*

	TOTAL FAT (GRAMS)	SATURATED FAT (GRAMS)	CALORIES
Breakfast			
Cold cereal (1 cup)	2.0	0.2	200
Banana (1)	0.6	0.1	105
Skim milk (1 cup)	0.4	0.3	86
Whole wheat bread (1 slice)	2.0	0.2	65
Margarine (½ tablespoon)	5.7	1.1	50
Fruit spread (1 tablespoon)	0.0	0.0	42
Snack			
Yoplait fat-free light yogurt (6 ounces)	0.0	0.0	90
Lunch			
Turkey sandwich:			
Turkey (w/o skin, 4 ounces)	2.7	0.8	133
Whole wheat bread (2 slices)	2.0	0.4	130
Lettuce (1 piece)	0.0	0.0	2
Tomato (2 slices)	0.1	0.0	8
Carrots, raw (2 medium)	0.3	0.0	62
Snack			
Oat bran muffin (1) *#1*	1.8	0.3	179
Warthog Dinner			
Pizza Hut supreme pan pizza (4 medium slices)	64.0	35.0	1260
Snack			
Orville Redenbacher Smart-Pop popcorn (6 cups)	2.0	2.0	100

Note: Recipe numbers follow dishes that appear in Resource 1.

Total fat: 83.6 grams (30%)   Saturated fat: 40.4 grams   Calories: 2512

Target 2400
Warthog Alternative #3

	TOTAL FAT (GRAMS)	SATURATED FAT (GRAMS)	CALORIES
Breakfast			
Cold cereal (1 cup)	2.0	0.2	200
Banana (1)	0.6	0.1	105
Skim milk (1 cup)	0.4	0.3	86
Whole wheat bread (1 slice)	2.0	0.2	65
Margarine (½ tablespoon)	5.7	1.1	50
Fruit spread (1 tablespoon)	0.0	0.0	42
Snack			
Yoplait fat-free light yogurt (6 ounces)	0.0	0.0	90
Lunch			
Turkey sandwich:			
Turkey (w/o skin, 4 ounces)	2.7	0.8	133
Whole wheat bread (2 slices)	2.0	0.4	130
Lettuce (1 piece)	0.0	0.0	2
Tomato (2 slices)	0.1	0.0	8
Carrots, raw (2 medium)	0.3	0.0	62
Snack			
Apple (1)	0.5	0.1	81
Warthog Dinner			
Kentucky Fried Chicken:			
Original Recipe chicken breast, wing, and drumstick	35.0	9.0	640
Biscuits (2)	24.0	3.2	400
Mashed potatoes	5.0	n/a	109
Coleslaw	6.0	n/a	114
Corn on the cob	12.0	n/a	222
Snack			
Orville Redenbacher Smart-Pop popcorn (6 cups)	2.0	2.0	100

Note: Recipe numbers follow dishes that appear in Resource 1.

Total fat: 89.3 grams (30%)   Saturated fat: 17.4 grams   Calories: 2639

Target 2400
Warthog Alternative #4

	TOTAL FAT (GRAMS)	SATURATED FAT (GRAMS)	CALORIES
Breakfast			
Cold cereal (1 cup)	2.0	0.2	200
Banana (1)	0.6	0.1	105
Skim milk (1 cup)	0.4	0.3	86
Whole wheat bread (1 slice)	2.0	0.2	65
Margarine (½ tablespoon)	5.7	1.1	50
Fruit spread (1 tablespoon)	0.0	0.0	42
Snack			
Yoplait fat-free light yogurt (6 ounces)	0.0	0.0	90
Lunch			
Turkey sandwich:			
Turkey (w/o skin, 4 ounces)	2.7	0.8	133
Whole wheat bread (2 slices)	2.0	0.4	130
Lettuce (1 piece)	0.0	0.0	2
Tomato (2 slices)	0.1	0.0	8
Carrots, raw (2 medium)	0.3	0.0	62
Snack			
Oat bran muffin (1) #1	1.8	0.3	179
Warthog Dinner			
Taco Bell bean burritos (2)	24.0	3.4	782
Taco Bell cinnamon twists (1 order)	6.0	2.0	139
Nachos	18.0	6.0	345
Snack			
Orville Redenbacher Smart-Pop popcorn (6 cups)	2.0	2.0	100

Note: Recipe numbers follow dishes that appear in Resource 1.

Total fat: 67.6 grams (24%)   Saturated fat: 16.8+ grams   Calories: 2518

Target 2400
Warthog Alternative #5

	TOTAL FAT (GRAMS)	SATURATED FAT (GRAMS)	CALORIES
Breakfast			
Cold cereal (½ cup)	1.0	0.1	100
Skim milk (½ cup)	0.2	0.1	43
Orange juice (1)	0.4	0.0	110
Snack			
Apple (1)	0.2	0.1	81
Wheat bran muffin (1) *#33*	2.1	0.5	177
Lunch			
Baked beans (½ cup) *#27*	1.5	0.3	208
Potato salad (½ cup) *#28*	3.5	0.5	166
Tomato (3 slices)	0.0	0.0	12
Snack			
Bagel (1)	1.0	0.1	200
Fat-free cream cheese (2 ounces)	0.0	0.0	50
Low-calorie cranberry juice (1 cup)	0.0	0.0	47
Warthog Dinner			
Pork loin chop, broiled (6 ounces)	43.0	15.6	602
Easy mashed potatoes (1 cup) *#29*	0.1	0.0	169
Carrots, cooked (½ cup)	0.1	0.0	24
Whole wheat bread (2 slices)	2.0	0.4	130
Healthy Choice low-fat ice cream (1 cup)	4.0	2.0	240
Low-fat hot fudge sauce (4 tablespoons)	2.0	0.0	180
Snack			
Mr. Phipps pretzels (12)	0.0	0.0	75

Note: Recipe numbers follow dishes that appear in Resource 1.

Total fat: 61.1 grams (21%)   Saturated fat: 19.7 grams   Calories: 2614

Resource 1
Jack Sprat Plan Recipes

1. OAT BRAN MUFFINS

Makes twelve muffins. Serving is one muffin.

2 egg whites or equivalent egg substitute
1 cup buttermilk
⅓ cup honey
⅓ cup molasses
2 cups oat bran
1⅔ cups whole wheat flour
2½ teaspoons baking soda
1½ to 2 cups fresh or frozen blueberries or other fruit

Beat egg whites lightly in bowl. Stir in buttermilk, honey, and molasses. In large bowl, stir together oat bran, flour, baking soda, and fruit. Add egg mixture and stir gently until all ingredients are blended.

Fill 12-cup nonstick or paper-lined muffin tin about ¾ full. Bake at 425 degrees about 15 minutes or until muffins test done. Let cool slightly. Remove from pans.

Total fat per serving: 1.8 grams   Saturated fat: 0.3 grams   Calories: 179

2. BROILED CODFISH

Makes four servings.

4 4-ounce (1 pound total) cod fillets
lemon juice
salt and pepper to taste

Place fish on rack coated with cooking spray; place rack on broiler pan. Broil 5½ inches from heat, 5 minutes each side or until fish flakes easily. Sprinkle with salt, pepper, and lemon juice.

Note: Other fish (4-ounce servings) with similar calories and fat content are sole, haddock, halibut, perch, and flounder. 4-ounce servings of salmon, tuna, and catfish have about 200 calories, 7 to 10 grams of fat, 1 to 2 grams of it saturated.

Total fat per serving: 1.0 grams   *Saturated fat: 0.2 grams*   *Calories: 118*

---

3. TARTAR SAUCE

Makes four servings.

½ cup fat-free plain yogurt
4 tablespoons fat-free salad dressing
4 tablespoons sweet pickle relish
2 teaspoons lemon juice
¼ teaspoon tarragon

Mix ingredients until blended well.

Total fat per serving: 0.1 grams   *Saturated fat: 0.0 grams*   *Calories: 28*

---

4. LARGE STUFFED PASTA SHELLS

Makes four servings.

12 jumbo pasta shells
1 pint light ricotta cheese
1 10-ounce package frozen chopped spinach, thawed and well-drained

1 cup fat-free mozzarella cheese, shredded
¼ cup Parmesan cheese
1 jar fat-free spaghetti sauce

Cook 12 pasta shells according to directions and drain. Cook spinach and squeeze as much liquid from it as possible. Combine spinach and cheeses. Stuff shells with spinach-cheese mixture. Cover bottom of 8 x 8-inch pan with ½ cup spaghetti sauce. Place stuffed shells in baking pan. Cover with remaining sauce. Bake 25-30 minutes at 350 degrees.

Total fat per serving: 4.8 grams   Saturated fat: 3.0 grams   Calories: 232

5. SALMON SALAD

Makes four servings.

8 ounces rigatoni, cooked and drained
2 medium cucumbers, peeled and chopped
8 small black olives
2 bunches romaine lettuce or 1 bunch romaine lettuce and 1 bunch
  fresh spinach, broken into bite-size pieces
1 14-ounce can salmon (tuna in spring water can be substituted)

DRESSING:

½ cup lemon juice
2 tablespoons basil
2 tablespoons honey
¼ teaspoon salt
2 teaspoons olive oil

Toss cooked rigatoni, cucumbers, olives, and lettuce. Mix dressing and pour over salad. Add salmon just before serving. This salad improves with age. Let it sit in the refrigerator overnight if you have time.

Total fat per serving: 9.7 grams   Saturated fat: 0.8 grams   Calories: 310

6. PARMESAN CHICKEN

Makes four servings.

4 chicken breasts
1 cup Parmesan cheese, grated
1 cup buttermilk

Preheat oven to 350 degrees. Coat chicken breasts with buttermilk, then Parmesan cheese. Place in baking dish. Bake 45 minutes.

Total fat per serving: 5.7 grams   Saturated fat: 2.6 grams   Calories: 199

7. TAPIOCA PUDDING

Makes three servings.

⅓ cup quick-cooking tapioca
2 tablespoons honey
3⅔ cups skim milk
2 egg whites
1 teaspoon vanilla (hazelnut flavoring is also good)

Whisk together tapioca, honey, milk, and egg whites in a deep bowl. Microwave uncovered for 13 minutes on high. Add flavoring. Stir and chill.

Total fat per serving: 0.4 grams   Saturated fat: 0.3 grams   Calories: 183

8. TUNA SALAD

Makes two servings.

1 6⅛-ounce can water-packed tuna
1 tablespoon Dijon mustard
2 tablespoons fat-free salad dressing
¼ cup celery
¼ cup sweet pickle relish

Drain tuna and mix with remaining ingredients.

Total fat per serving: 2.7 grams   Saturated fat: 0.6 grams   Calories: 171

9. STIR-FRY VEGETABLES WITH CHICKEN

Makes four servings.

1 cup fresh broccoli, chopped
1 cup fresh cauliflower, chopped
1 cup fresh carrots, chopped
1 cup fresh onions, chopped
1 cup fresh mushrooms, chopped
1 6-ounce package frozen snow peas
3 cups chicken, diced and cooked
¼ cup low-sodium soy sauce

Stir-fry vegetables in small amount of water. Add cooked chicken and heat thoroughly. Serve over brown rice with low-sodium soy sauce.

Total fat per serving: 11 grams   *Saturated fat: 2.1 grams*   *Calories: 261*

10. CHEF SALAD

Makes three servings.

4 cups lettuce, cut into bite-size pieces
½ cup mushrooms, sliced
3 carrots, sliced
½ cup cauliflower, chopped
1 green pepper, diced
½ cup turkey, cut in strips
2 tomatoes, sliced
½ cup low-fat cheddar cheese, shredded

Toss lettuce, mushrooms, carrots, cauliflower, and green pepper. Arrange strips of turkey and tomato slices on top. Sprinkle with cheese. Serve with low-calorie dressing.

Total fat per serving: 7.0 grams   *Saturated fat: 3.9 grams*   *Calories: 156*

11. POPPYSEED DRESSING

Makes four servings.

1 cup fat-free plain yogurt
2 tablespoons maple syrup
2 teaspoons poppyseeds
¼ teaspoon salt

Stir ingredients together until mixture is smooth. Serve chilled.

Total fat per serving: 0.2 grams   Saturated fat: 0.0 grams   Calories: 54

---

12. MULTI-GRAIN PANCAKES

Makes twelve pancakes. Serving is two pancakes.

⅔ cup whole wheat flour
⅔ cup all-purpose flour
¼ cup oat bran
2 tablespoons wheat germ
1 teaspoon baking powder
½ teaspoon baking soda
¼ teaspoon salt
1 cup buttermilk
2 teaspoons honey
¼ cup skim milk
2 egg whites
1 tablespoon unsweetened applesauce
¼ teaspoon vanilla (optional)

Mix dry ingredients together in medium bowl. In second bowl, combine buttermilk, honey, skim milk, egg whites, applesauce, and vanilla; add to dry ingredients. Mix together until dry ingredients are moist. Heat a griddle or skillet sprayed with cooking oil at medium.
    Pour ¼ cup of batter onto griddle or skillet. Turn heat to medium low. Cook pancakes until tops begin to bubble. Flip pancakes over and cook until golden brown.

Total fat per serving: 8.0 grams   Saturated fat: 1.6 grams   Calories: 324

---

13. SHRIMP FETTUCINE

Makes four servings.

12 ounces frozen or fresh shrimp, peeled and deveined
1 teaspoon cajun seasoning
1 clove garlic, minced
½ cup onion, chopped
2 carrots, sliced
1 cup broccoli, chopped
1 cup mushrooms, chopped
1 cup zucchini, chopped
¼ cup Parmesan cheese, grated
1 cup skim milk
4 cups fettucine, cooked

Lightly spray a medium-sized skillet with cooking oil. Place shrimp, cajun seasoning, and garlic in skillet and cook over medium heat until shrimp turns pink. Add vegetables and cover pan. Cook vegetables until they reach desired doneness. Add Parmesan cheese and milk, stirring until cheese melts. Add pasta, stir together and cook 1 to 2 minutes.

Total fat per serving: 7.1 grams   Saturated fat: 3.2 grams   Calories: 425

14. RED BEANS AND RICE

Makes four servings.

1 medium green pepper, chopped
1 spear celery, chopped
½ cup onion, chopped
1 clove garlic, minced
1 teaspoon oregano
1 teaspoon cayenne pepper
½ teaspoon black pepper
2 cups canned red beans
2 cups brown rice, cooked

Sauté green pepper, celery, and onion slowly in small amount of water to keep from sticking. Add remaining ingredients and simmer until heated through.

Total fat per serving: 1.7 grams   Saturated fat: 0.3 grams   Calories: 229

---

15. LOW-FAT CHEESE SAUCE

Makes four servings.

½ cup all-purpose flour
2 cups skim milk
½ cup low-fat cheddar cheese, shredded
3 teaspoons chives or green onions, chopped
1 teaspoon paprika

Stir flour and cold milk in saucepan until smooth. Cook over medium heat, stirring constantly, until bubbly and thickened. Add cheese and chives or onions, stirring until cheese melts. Sprinkle with paprika.

Total fat per serving: 2.4 grams   Saturated fat: 1.4 grams   Calories: 121

---

16. CHICKEN WITH DIJON MUSTARD

Makes four servings

4 skinless, boned chicken breasts
½ cup Dijon mustard
2 tablespoons honey
3 tablespoons lemon juice

Preheat oven to 350 degrees. Mix mustard, honey, and lemon juice. Place chicken in shallow baking pan. Set aside ¼ cup sauce. Pour remaining sauce on chicken. Cover and bake 20 minutes. Uncover and bake another 10 minutes or until done. Remove chicken to serving plate. Mix reserved sauce with sauce in pan; then pour over chicken.

Total fat per serving: 4.9 grams   Saturated fat: 0.9 grams   Calories: 205

17. LENTIL SALAD WITH TOMATOES AND RICE

Makes four servings.

1 cup lentils, cooked and drained
1 16-ounce can tomatoes, diced
1½ cups brown rice
1 cucumber, seeded and diced
1 teaspoon oregano
1 tablespoon vinegar
1 teaspoon olive oil
½ cup scallions
2 teaspoons lemon juice
salt and pepper, if desired

Mix ingredients together. Can be served warmed or chilled.

Total fat per serving: 0.6 grams   Saturated fat: 0.1 grams   Calories: 65

18. VEGETABLE MEDLEY

Makes four servings.

1 potato, unpeeled and diced small
1½ cups zucchini, sliced thin
2 green peppers, diced
1 medium onion, chopped
1 medium eggplant, unpeeled and diced
1 cup garbanzo beans
1 tablespoon olive oil
1 teaspoon salt
¼ teaspoon pepper
4 large tomatoes, sliced
2 tablespoons vinegar
3 teaspoons basil
3 teaspoons parsley

In large bowl, mix potato, zucchini, peppers, onion, eggplant, and beans with olive oil, basil, parsley, salt, and pepper. Place half the mixture in an oiled 3-quart casserole. Top with half the tomato slices. Add remaining mixture and top with other half of tomato slices. Pour vinegar over top. Cover and bake at 350 degrees for 1½ hours. Serve hot or cold.

Total fat per serving: 4.2 grams   *Saturated fat: 0.6*   *Calories: 126*

19. GRILLED CHEESE

Makes one sandwich.

2 slices whole wheat bread
2 slices fat-free cheese
1 tablespoon margarine

Make sandwich. Spread margarine on both sides of sandwich and grill in skillet.

Total fat per serving: 8.0 grams   *Saturated fat: 1.6 grams*   *Calories: 260*

20. BROCCOLI-RICE CASSEROLE

Makes five servings.

2 cups brown rice
2 cups broccoli, chopped
1 cup onion, chopped
¼ cup Parmesan cheese, grated
1 cup fat-free cottage cheese

Prepare rice as directed. Sauté broccoli and onion. Combine ingredients. Bake 20-25 minutes at 350 degrees or until heated through. Can be microwaved.

Total fat per serving: 5.3 grams   Saturated fat: 2.9 grams   Calories: 221

21. WHITE BEAN CHILI

Makes eight servings.

1 cup onion, chopped
2 cloves garlic, minced
6 cups water
16 ounces dry white beans, rinsed
1 potato, diced
1 4-ounce can green chilies, chopped
2 teaspoons chili powder
1 teaspoon cumin
1 teaspoon oregano
2 cups chicken, diced and cooked

Sauté onion and garlic slowly, using a small amount of water, if necessary, to keep from sticking. Add water, beans, potato, green chilies, and spices. Bring to a boil, then simmer about 3 hours until beans are tender. Add cooked chicken last 30 minutes of cooking time.

Total fat per serving: 2.9 grams   Saturated fat: 0.7 grams   Calories: 235

22. VEGETABLE LASAGNA

Makes eight servings.

1½ cups onions, chopped
2 cloves garlic, minced
½ cup mushrooms, sliced
4 cups broccoli, chopped
2 cups spinach, torn in small pieces
1 cup fat-free mozzarella cheese, shredded
½ cup Parmesan cheese, grated
¼ cup parsley, chopped
½ teaspoon pepper
½ teaspoon salt
3 cups fat-free spaghetti sauce
8 ounces whole wheat lasagna noodles

In a large skillet, sauté onions, garlic, and mushrooms until tender, cooking slowly to prevent sticking. Add broccoli and spinach. Cook until broccoli is crisp-tender. In medium bowl, combine cheeses, parsley, pepper, and salt. Place ½ cup spaghetti sauce on bottom of 13 x 9-inch baking pan. Layer lasagna noodles, spread ½ cheese mixture over noodles, then ½ vegetable mixture, then ½ remaining sauce. Repeat layers and place lasagna noodles on top. Cover top with remaining sauce. Bake at 375 degrees for 30 minutes. Let cool slightly before cutting.

Total fat per serving: 6.9 grams   Saturated fat: 3.6 grams   Calories: 300

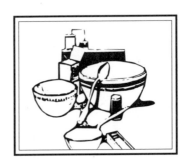

23. POTATO SOUP

Makes six servings.

4 medium potatoes, peeled and cubed
1 onion, chopped
2 tablespoons flour
1 teaspoon thyme
1 teaspoon salt
½ teaspoon pepper
1 teaspoon marjoram
2 tablespoons parsley, chopped
2 cups hot potato water
3 cups skim milk

In saucepan, cover potatoes and onion with water and cook until potatoes are tender. Drain potatoes and onion, saving liquid. In saucepan, stir flour into 1 cup cold milk. When blended, add potato liquid and rest of milk. Stir spices and parsley into liquid. Cook over medium heat until soup thickens slightly. Stir in potatoes and onions. Heat through.

Total fat per serving: 0.4 grams   *Saturated fat: 0.2*   *Calories: 133*

24. PITA POCKET WITH VEGETABLES

Makes one serving.

1 whole wheat pita pocket
1 thin slice of onion
1 slice of fresh tomato
1 slice fat-free cheese
¼ cup sprouts
2 slices green pepper
¼ cup zucchini, sliced
1 tablespoon Dijon mustard

Spread mustard on inside of pita pocket. Stuff pita with cheese and vegetables.

Total fat per serving: 2.2 grams   *Saturated fat: 0.1 grams*   *Calories: 209*

25. SPINACH MUSHROOM LASAGNA

Makes six servings.

16 ounces whole wheat lasagna noodles, uncooked
4 cups fresh spinach
2 cups fat-free cottage cheese
2 egg whites
½ cup fresh mushrooms, sliced
1 20-ounce jar fat-free spaghetti sauce

Preheat oven to 350 degrees. Combine cottage cheese and egg whites. Mix mushrooms with spaghetti sauce. Pour ½ cup of sauce in bottom of 12 x 7-inch pan. Cover with a layer of noodles (the noodles will cook in the oven). Spread with cottage cheese mixture. Layer spinach leaves on top of cottage cheese. Cover with half of remaining sauce. Make another layer with the cottage cheese, spinach, and sauce, saving about ½ cup of the sauce for the top. Place last layer of noodles on top and cover with remaining sauce. Bake 1 hour. Let cool slightly before cutting.

Total fat per serving: 1.0 grams	*Saturated fat: 0.0*	*Calories: 235*

26. EGGPLANT PARMESAN WITH PASTA

Makes four servings.

1 large or 2 small eggplants
salt
8 ounces ziti
1 clove garlic, minced
1⅓ cups fat-free cottage cheese
½ cup Parmesan cheese, grated
1 tablespoon parsley
½ teaspoon basil
½ teaspoon oregano
2 cups fat-free spaghetti sauce

Cut eggplant into ¼-inch slices and sprinkle with salt. Let salted eggplant drain in colander for 30 minutes (this removes the bitter juices from the eggplant).

Cook ziti and drain. Preheat oven to 400 degrees.

Rinse eggplant well with water; then rub with garlic. Broil eggplant 4 inches from heat about 2 minutes each side or place eggplant in microwave on high for 3 minutes.

In a large bowl, combine cottage cheese, Parmesan cheese, parsley, basil, and oregano, and toss with ziti.

Spread a thin layer of spaghetti sauce on the bottom of a 2½- to 3-quart casserole, add half the ziti mixture, then half the eggplant slices, then half the remaining sauce. Repeat the three layers. Cover and bake for 30 minutes. Remove cover and bake another 15 minutes or until the top is lightly browned.

Total fat per serving: 6.9 grams   Saturated fat: 3.7 grams   Calories: 300

27. BAKED BEANS

Makes eight servings.

4 cups canned baked beans, approximately 32 ounces
1 cup barbecue sauce
3 tablespoons Dijon mustard
2 tablespoons Worcestershire sauce
½ cup brown sugar, packed

Mix all ingredients well. Place in casserole and bake at 300 degrees for 2 hours.

Total fat per serving: 1.5 grams   Saturated fat: 0.3 grams   Calories: 208

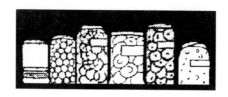

28. POTATO SALAD

Makes six servings.

5 medium potatoes
1 cup celery, sliced
1 cup onion, chopped
3 teaspoons dill weed
½ cup sweet pickle relish
1 cup fat-free sour cream
½ cup light mayonnaise

In large pan, cover potatoes with water and cook over medium heat until tender, adding water if necessary. Drain potatoes, let cool. Dice potatoes, leaving skin on if desired. Mix all ingredients together. Chill until ready to serve.

Total fat per serving: 7.0 grams   Saturated fat: 1.0 grams   Calories: 332

29. EASY, HEALTHY MASHED POTATOES

Makes four servings.

6 medium potatoes, peeled and diced
¼ cup skim milk
1¼ cups fat-free plain yogurt
4 green onions, sliced
salt and pepper to taste

Place potatoes in microwave-safe dish. Add milk. Cover tightly. Cook on high until potatoes are tender but not mushy (about 12 minutes). Remove from microwave. Add yogurt and onions. Mash together. Season to taste with salt and pepper.

Total fat per serving: 0.2 grams   Saturated fat: 0.1 grams   Calories: 169

30. CINNAMON-RAISIN BISCUITS

Makes twelve biscuits. Serving is one biscuit.

¼ cup sugar
1 teaspoon cinnamon
2 cups all-purpose flour
2 teaspoons baking powder
½ teaspoon baking soda
½ teaspoon salt
4 tablespoons margarine
1 cup fat-free plain yogurt
½ cup seedless raisins
½ cup confectioner's sugar
1 to 2 teaspoons water or orange juice

Preheat oven to 450 degrees. In a small bowl, mix sugar and cinnamon. In a large bowl, combine half the sugar-cinnamon mixture with flour, baking powder, baking soda, and salt. Cut margarine into flour mixture until crumbly. Make well in center of flour mixture. Add yogurt and raisins, stirring just until dough clings together. On a lightly floured surface, knead dough gently 8 to 10 times. Roll dough to ½-inch thickness. Cut with 2½-inch biscuit cutter.

Place biscuits on ungreased baking sheet. Sprinkle with the remaining sugar-cinnamon mixture. Bake for 10 to 12 minutes or until golden brown. Remove from baking sheet and cool slightly on wire racks.

Combine confectioner's sugar and water or juice to make icing. Drizzle over biscuits while warm.

Total fat per serving: 4.0 grams   Saturated fat: 0.7 grams   Calories: 166

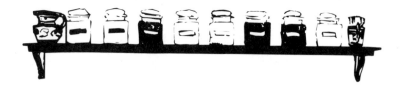

31. CARROT-OATMEAL COOKIES

Makes three to four dozen cookies. Serving is two cookies.

½ cup unsweetened applesauce
⅓ cup brown sugar
⅓ cup molasses
1 egg white or equivalent egg substitute
1 cup all-purpose flour
½ teaspoon baking powder
½ teaspoon baking soda
1 teaspoon nutmeg
¼ cup powdered milk
1 teaspoon salt
1 teaspoon cinnamon
1 cup carrot, shredded
½ cup seedless raisins
1¼ cups rolled oats

Preheat oven to 400 degrees. In a large bowl, mix together apple-sauce, brown sugar, molasses, and egg. In separate bowl, sift together flour, baking powder, baking soda, nutmeg, dry milk, salt, and cinnamon. Add flour mixture to applesauce mixture. Add carrots, raisins, and oats to flour mixture. Mix well. Drop the dough by rounded teaspoons about 2 inches apart on lightly oiled baking sheets. Bake for about 10 minutes, until lightly browned around the edges. Place cookies on rack to cool.

Total fat per serving: 0.9 grams   Saturated fat: 0.1 grams   Calories: 110

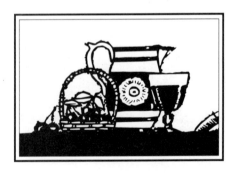

32. CHEESE AND NOODLES

Makes four servings.

8 ounces noodles, cooked and drained
1 clove garlic, minced
1 cup spinach, cooked
2 teaspoons basil
2 tablespoons parsley
1 cup fat-free ricotta cheese or fat-free cottage cheese
2 tablespoons Parmesan cheese, grated
salt and pepper to taste

In 10-inch skillet, sauté garlic and spinach for 5 minutes. Add basil, parsley, ricotta cheese, salt, and pepper. Stir mixture until blended and heated through. Combine the spinach-cheese mixture and the noodles. Sprinkle Parmesan cheese on top.

Total fat per serving: 3.3 grams   Saturated fat: 1.5 grams   Calories: 301

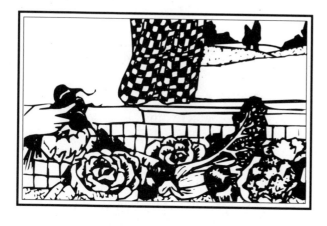

33. WHEAT BRAN MUFFINS

Makes twelve muffins. Serving is one muffin.

½ stick light margarine
⅔ cup honey
2 egg whites or equivalent egg substitute
1¼ cups buttermilk
⅔ cup whole wheat flour
1 cup all-purpose flour
2 cups wheat bran
¼ teaspoon salt
2 teaspoons baking soda
1 cup seedless raisins or other fruit
   (drained if canned; blueberries included in grocery list as option)

Melt margarine and mix with honey, eggs, and buttermilk, beating to combine completely. Add flours, wheat bran, salt, and baking soda and stir lightly to blend. If consistency is runny, add more flour. Add raisins or other fruit as desired. Prepare muffin tin (use paper liners or spray lightly with cooking spray). Bake at 350 degrees for 30 minutes or until the muffins are done. Let cool slightly, then remove from pan and allow to cool on rack.

Total fat per serving: 2.1 grams   Saturated fat: 0.5 grams   Calories: 177

---

34. BROWN RICE WITH BLACK-EYED PEAS

Makes four servings.

1 15-ounce can black-eyed peas
1 15-ounce can diced tomatoes with chili seasoning
2 cups brown rice

Cook rice according to package directions in two-quart microwave bowl. Add black-eyed peas and diced tomatoes to rice and heat in microwave on high 4-5 minutes until peas and tomatoes are heated.

Total fat per serving: 1.9 grams   Saturated fat: 0.2   Calories: 222

---

35. SPICY BARBECUE CHICKEN

Makes four servings.

¼ cup barbecue sauce
2 tablespoons ketchup
1 tablespoon honey
1 tablespoon red wine vinegar
1 tablespoon ground ginger
1 tablespoon Dijon mustard
¾ teaspoon black pepper
1 clove garlic
½ teaspoon cayenne pepper
4 skinless chicken breasts

Mix ingredients (except chicken) together well. Use to baste chicken breasts while grilling or baking. Grill about 10 minutes each side until meat is no longer pink, or bake at 350 degrees for 30 minutes or until done.

Total fat per serving: 3.6 grams   *Saturated fat: 1.0 grams*   *Calories: 178*

36. GREEN BEANS AND RICE

Makes four servings.

2 cups brown rice
2 cups fresh green beans
½ cup onion, diced
2 teaspoons olive oil
1 clove garlic, minced
1 tablespoon dill

Cook rice following package directions. Wash beans, and snap off ends if desired. Set aside. Sauté diced onion in oil until soft. Add garlic. Cook for 1 minute. Stir in dill and green beans. Cook over high heat until beans are bright green and tender. Stir often. Layer beans with rice in casserole and cover. Bake at 350 degrees for 10 to 15 minutes.

Total fat per serving: 2.9 grams   *Saturated fat: 0.5 grams*   *Calories: 157*

37. PASTA PRIMAVERA

Makes four servings.

1 cup carrots, thinly sliced
1 large clove garlic, minced
1 14½-ounce can stewed tomatoes
1 cup mushrooms, sliced
2 tablespoons cornstarch
2 teaspoons basil, crushed
½ teaspoon oregano, crushed
1 16-ounce can cut green beans
8 ounces rigatoni, cooked and drained
¼ cup Parmesan cheese, grated
1 tablespoon parsley

Sauté carrots and garlic in small amount of water over medium-low heat until carrots are tender-crisp (about five minutes). Stir in tomatoes, mushrooms, cornstarch, basil, and oregano. Cook, stirring constantly until sauce is thickened and translucent. Add beans and heat through. Add pasta to skillet; toss with cheese. Garnish with parsley.

Total fat per serving: 3.9 grams   Saturated fat: 1.6 grams   Calories: 336

38. VEGGIE CHILI

Makes four servings.

1½ cups zucchini, cubed
1 cup onions, chopped
2 cloves garlic, minced
1 medium green pepper, diced
2 cups canned or fresh tomatoes
3 teaspoons chili powder
1½ teaspoons oregano
⅓ cup fresh parsley
salt and pepper to taste
2 cups canned kidney beans, approximately 16 ounces

Sauté zucchini, onion, garlic, and green pepper in large saucepan for 10 minutes until vegetables are softened. Add tomatoes, chili powder, oregano, parsley, salt, and pepper. Cook over low heat, uncovered for 10 minutes. Stir in beans and cook 10 minutes more on low heat.

Total fat per serving: 1.1 grams   Saturated fat: 0.2 grams   Calories: 193

---

39. LINGUINE WITH VEGETABLES

Makes four servings.

1 16-ounce package of linguine
3 cups cauliflower, cut in bite-size pieces
4 cups broccoli, cut in bite-size pieces
2 tablespoons all-purpose flour
1½ teaspoons instant chicken bouillon
1 teaspoon salt
2½ cups skim milk
¼ cup Parmesan cheese, grated
¼ cup pine nuts, toasted (optional)

Prepare linguine according to package directions. Drain. Keep linguine warm in pan while preparing vegetables. Steam cauliflower and broccoli until tender but still crisp. While vegetables are cooking, in 2-quart saucepan over medium heat, add flour, chicken bouillon, and salt with small amount milk. Stir constantly for 1 minute. Gradually add rest of milk, stirring until mixture thickens. Remove saucepan from heat; stir in Parmesan cheese until sauce is smooth.

To serve, toss linguine, broccoli, and cauliflower. Place mixture on plates and serve with sauce. Top with pine nuts, if desired.

Total fat per serving: 6.4 grams   Saturated fat: 2.4 grams   Calories: 285

---

40. LOW-FAT CHEESECAKE

Makes twelve servings.

4 cups (1 32-ounce carton) plain fat-free yogurt
1½ cups graham cracker crumbs
2 cups fat-free ricotta cheese
1 cup fat-free sour cream
¾ cup honey
4 tablespoons cornstarch
5 egg whites
2 teaspoons flavoring
(hazelnut, lemon, amaretto, or vanilla can be used)
1 tablespoon margarine

Drain whey from yogurt by placing yogurt in cheesecloth-lined colander. Place colander in large bowl to catch whey. Allow to drain about 24 hours. Discard the whey.

Melt margarine and mix with graham cracker crumbs. Preheat oven to 300 degrees. With a spoon or your fingertips, press graham cracker crumbs in bottom and slightly up sides of 9-inch springform pan. Mix yogurt cheese, ricotta cheese, sour cream, honey, cornstarch, egg whites, and flavoring until smooth. Pour into graham cracker crust. Bake 60-75 minutes until center is set and cheesecake is lightly browned around the edges. Cool, refrigerate until thoroughly chilled. Serve as is or top with your favorite fresh fruit.

Total fat per serving: 3.1 grams   Saturated fat: 0.7 grams   Calories: 268

---

41. MUSHROOM-BARLEY SOUP

Makes six servings.

3 cups mushrooms, sliced
1 cup onion, chopped
½ cup leek, chopped
6 cups water
4 teaspoons instant chicken bouillon or bouillon cubes
2 large potatoes, peeled and sliced
1 cup carrots, sliced

½ cup barley
3 bay leaves

Separate mushroom stems from caps. Chop stems. Slice caps and set aside. In large saucepan, sauté mushroom stems, onion, and leek until tender. (Add a small amount of water if necessary to prevent sticking.) Stir in chicken broth, potatoes, carrots, barley, and bay leaves. Cover pan and simmer 30 minutes. Uncover; add sliced mushroom caps and continue simmering until vegetables are tender, about 25 minutes. Season to taste with salt and pepper.

Total fat per serving: 0.4 grams   Saturated fat: 0.1 grams   Calories: 85

42. POUND CAKE

Makes twelve servings.

½ cup unsweetened applesauce
½ cup skim milk
1 teaspoon vanilla
3½ teaspoons almond extract
2¾ cups all-purpose flour
2 teaspoons baking powder
8 egg whites
1¼ cups granulated sugar

Combine applesauce, skim milk, vanilla, and almond extract. Mix flour and baking powder. Add to applesauce mixture. Beat egg whites until foamy, gradually adding sugar to egg whites until stiff peaks form. Gently fold mixture together. Oil and flour a tube pan. Bake at 350 degrees for 50-55 minutes. Invert immediately. Cool. Good served with fresh strawberries.

Total fat per serving: 0.3 grams   Saturated fat: 0.1 grams   Calories: 235

43. PEANUT BUTTER SANDWICH

Makes one sandwich.

2 slices whole wheat bread
2 tablespoons peanut butter
2 tablespoons fruit spread

Total fat per serving: 18.4 grams   Saturated fat: 3.2 grams   Calories: 386

44. PASTA SALAD WITH TUNA

Makes four servings.

½ cup fat-free plain yogurt
1½ teaspoons honey
1 tablespoon lemon juice
1 teaspoon dill
¼ teaspoon celery seed
¼ teaspoon paprika
1½ cups pasta shells or spirals, cooked
1 6½-ounce can water-packed tuna
½ cup peas
½ cup celery, chopped
¼ cup green pepper, diced
2 tablespoons green onion, chopped

Mix yogurt, honey, lemon juice, vinegar, dill, celery seed, and paprika in large bowl. Stir in pasta, tuna, peas, celery, and pepper. Toss gently to thoroughly coat ingredients with dressing. Garnish with green onion. Serve at room temperature. If chilled, let sit at room temperature about 15 minutes before serving.

Total fat per serving: 1.7 grams   Saturated fat: 0.4 grams   Calories: 210

45. LENTIL CASSEROLE

Makes six servings.

1 cup onion, chopped
¾ cup lentils, uncooked
¾ cup brown rice, uncooked
3 ounces low-fat cheddar cheese, grated
½ teaspoon thyme
½ teaspoon basil
½ teaspoon oregano
½ teaspoon salt
½ teaspoon garlic powder
2 10½-ounce cans fat-free chicken broth

Coat 1½-quart casserole with cooking spray. Mix everything together in casserole. Cover and bake at 350 degrees for 1½ hours or until lentils are tender.

Total fat per serving: 2.4 grams   Saturated fat: 1.0 grams   Calories: 141

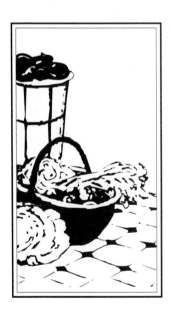

46. CARROT CAKE

Makes eight servings.

1½ teaspoons baking soda
¼ cup warm water
1½ cups carrots, shredded
½ cup fat-free plain yogurt
¾ cup sugar
¾ cup unsweetened applesauce
1 egg white
2 teaspoons cinnamon
½ teaspoon nutmeg
½ teaspoon cloves, ground
½ teaspoon salt
1 cup seedless raisins
1 cup whole wheat flour
1 cup all-purpose flour

Preheat oven to 325 degrees. In small bowl, combine baking soda and warm water. Set aside. In a large bowl, combine carrots, yogurt, sugar, applesauce, egg white, cinnamon, nutmeg, cloves, salt, and raisins. Stir in whole-wheat flour and all-purpose flour; then stir in the reserved baking-soda mixture. Pour the batter into a lightly greased 9-inch square baking pan. Bake for 1 hour or until cake tests done. Let cake cool in pan on a rack for 10 minutes before removing.

Total fat per serving: 0.8 grams   Saturated fat: 0.2 grams   Calories: 262

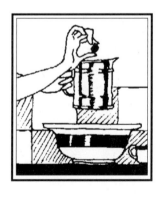

47. BUTTERMILK CHICKEN

Makes four servings.

4 skinless chicken breasts
3 or 4 cups buttermilk
salt and pepper to taste

Place chicken in bowl. Pour buttermilk over breasts. Cover bowl and refrigerate overnight, turning chicken occasionally. When ready to cook, preheat oven to 400 degrees. Remove chicken from buttermilk marinade and place on rack in pan. Season with salt and pepper. Bake until done, approximately 45 minutes. If meat is browning too quickly, cover lightly with foil.

Total fat per serving: 3.5 grams   Saturated fat: 1.2 grams   Calories: 175

48. MIXED VEGETABLES

Makes four servings.

½ cup carrots, sliced
½ cup broccoli, chopped
½ cup cauliflower, chopped
2 tablespoons Dijon mustard
2 tablespoons honey
1 teaspoon dill

Steam carrots for 10 minutes. Add broccoli and cauliflower. Steam until tender, about 8 more minutes. Mix together mustard, honey, and dill to make a smooth sauce. Pour sauce over vegetables and mix.

Total fat per serving: 0.4 gram   Saturated fat: 0.0 grams   Calories: 51

49. BEAN BURRITOS

Makes 1 serving (2 burritos).

2 flour tortillas
½ cup fat-free vegetarian refried beans
¼ cup salsa

Warm tortillas in oven. Place half the refried beans on each tortilla. Add salsa and roll tortillas around mixture. Add onions if desired.

Total fat per serving: 6.4 grams   Saturated fat: 0.8 grams   Calories: 290

50. OVEN CRISPY FISH

Makes four servings.

2 cups fat-free cracker or bread crumbs
¼ teaspoon dry mustard
1 egg white
2 tablespoons skim milk
4 4-ounce (1 pound total) fish fillets of choice
lemon wedges

Preheat oven to 425 degrees. Stir mustard into bread crumbs. Beat egg white and milk in bowl for dipping fillets. Spread cracker crumbs on a plate. Dip fish in egg white mixture, then coat with cracker crumbs. Place on baking sheet. Bake for about 15 minutes, until coating is crisp and fish flakes easily with a fork. Serve with lemon wedges.

Total fat per serving: 1.7 grams   Saturated fat: 0.5 grams   Calories: 166

51. APPLE BREAD

Makes two loaves, ten slices each.

¼ cup honey
½ cup unsweetened applesauce
¼ cup orange juice
8 ounces egg substitute

4 cups all-purpose flour
¾ cup sugar
1 teaspoon salt
1 teaspoon baking soda
2 teaspoons baking powder
1 tablespoon vanilla
2 Granny Smith apples, unpeeled and chopped
2 cups seedless raisins
¼ cup buttermilk

Preheat oven to 350 degrees. In large bowl, mix honey, buttermilk, applesauce, orange juice, and egg substitute together. In another large bowl, mix flour, sugar, salt, baking soda, and baking powder. Gradually mix flour mixture into egg mixture until well blended. Add vanilla, chopped apples, and raisins. Spray two bread pans with cooking oil. Place half of the bread batter in each. Bake 1 hour or until done. Let bread cool in pan a few minutes; then turn onto wire rack to cool completely.

Total fat per serving: 0.8 gram   Saturated fat: 0.2 grams   Calories: 193

---

52. SALMON WITH ZUCCHINI AND MUSHROOMS

Makes four servings.

1 pound salmon
1 medium zucchini, sliced
½ cup mushrooms, sliced
1 tablespoon dill
¼ cup dry white wine

Preheat oven to 450 degrees. Spray bottom of pan or casserole with cooking oil. Place salmon on bottom of baking dish, with zucchini, mushrooms, dill, and wine on top. Cover and bake 12 to 15 minutes until done.

Total fat per serving: 8.6 grams   Saturated fat: 1.6 grams   Calories: 228

Resource 2

Substitution Tables

	TOTAL FAT (GRAMS)	SATURATED FAT (GRAMS)	CALORIES
Breakfast and Snack			
Apple bread #51	0.8	0.2	193
Oat bran muffins #1	1.8	0.3	179
Wheat bran muffins #33	2.1	0.5	177
Cinnamon-raisin biscuits #30	4.0	0.7	166
Multi-grain pancakes #12	8.0	1.6	323
Lunch and Dinner			
Peanut butter sandwich #43	18.4	3.2	386
Easy mashed potatoes #29	0.2	0.1	169
Potato soup #23	0.4	0.2	133
Mushroom-barley soup #41	0.4	0.1	85
Mixed vegetables #48	0.4	0.0	51
Lentil salad #17	0.6	0.1	65
Spinach mushroom lasagna #25	1.0	0.0	235
Broiled codfish #2	1.0	0.2	118
Veggie chili #38	1.1	0.2	193
Red beans and rice #14	1.7	0.3	229
Pasta salad with tuna #44	1.7	0.4	210
Oven crispy fish #50	1.7	0.5	166
Brown rice with black-eyed peas #34	1.9	0.2	222

	TOTAL FAT (GRAMS)	SATURATED FAT (GRAMS)	CALORIES
Pita with veggies *#24*	2.2	0.1	209
Tuna salad *#8*	2.7	0.6	171
White bean chili *#21*	2.9	0.7	235
Green beans and rice *#36*	2.9	0.5	157
Baked beans *#27*	1.5	0.3	208
Cheese and noodles *#32*	3.3	1.5	301
Buttermilk chicken *#47*	3.5	1.2	175
Spicy barbecue chicken *#35*	3.6	1.0	178
Lentil casserole *#45*	2.4	1.0	141
Pasta primavera *#37*	3.9	1.6	336
Vegetable medley *#18*	4.2	0.6	126
Large stuffed pasta shells *#4*	4.8	3.0	232
Chicken with Dijon mustard *#16*	4.9	0.9	205
Broccoli-rice casserole *#20*	5.3	2.9	221
Parmesan chicken *#6*	5.7	2.6	199
Linguine with vegetables *#39*	6.4	2.4	285
Bean burritos *#49*	6.4	0.8	290
Eggplant Parmesan with pasta *#26*	6.9	3.7	300
Vegetable lasagna *#22*	6.9	3.6	300
Chef salad *#10*	7.0	3.9	156
Shrimp fettucine *#13*	7.1	3.2	425
Potato salad *#28*	7.0	1.0	332
Grilled cheese *#19*	8.0	1.6	260
Salmon with zucchini and mushrooms *#52*	8.6	1.6	228
Salmon salad *#5*	9.7	0.8	310
Stir-fry vegetables with chicken *#9*	11.0	2.1	261

Desserts

	TOTAL FAT (GRAMS)	SATURATED FAT (GRAMS)	CALORIES
Pound cake *#42*	0.3	0.1	235
Tapioca pudding *#7*	0.4	0.3	183
Carrot cake *#46*	0.8	0.2	262
Carrot-oatmeal cookies *#31*	0.9	0.1	110
Low-fat cheesecake *#40*	3.1	0.7	268

Sauces and Dressings

	TOTAL FAT (GRAMS)	SATURATED FAT (GRAMS)	CALORIES
Tartar sauce *#3*	0.1	0.0	28
Poppyseed dressing *#11*	0.2	0.0	54
Low-fat cheese sauce *#15*	2.4	1.4	121

Resource 3

Fast Food Choices

	TOTAL FAT (GRAMS)	SATURATED FAT (GRAMS)	CALORIES
Breakfast			
Arby's			
Blueberry muffin	7.0	2.0	240
Hardee's			
Three pancakes	2.0	1.0	280
Three pancakes, 2 bacon strips	9.0	3.0	350
Bagel, plain	3.0	0.0	200
McDonald's			
Fat-free apple bran muffin	<1.0	0.0	180
English muffin	2.0	0.0	140
Wheaties	1.0	0.0	80
Cheerios	1.0	0.0	70
Hotcakes	4.0	n/a	280
Lunch and Dinner			
Arby's			
Old fashioned chicken noodle soup	2.0	n/a	99
Plain baked potato	2.0	0.0	240

	TOTAL FAT (GRAMS)	SATURATED FAT (GRAMS)	CALORIES
Arby's (cont'd)			
Lumberjack mixed vegetable soup	4.0	n/a	89
Roast turkey deluxe	6.0	n/a	260
Roast chicken salad	7.0	n/a	204
Roast chicken deluxe	7.0	n/a	276
Cream of broccoli soup	7.0	n/a	166
Potato bacon soup	9.0	n/a	184
Roast beef deluxe	10.0	n/a	294
Chef salad	10.0	n/a	205
Garden salad	5.0	n/a	117
Boston clam chowder	10.0	n/a	193
Junior roast beef	11.0	3.0	233
Light Italian dressing	1.0	n/a	23
Burger King			
Broiled chicken salad	10.0	n/a	200
Garden salad	5.0	0.0	95
Hamburger	10.0	n/a	260
Captain D's			
Chicken dinner	8.0	n/a	414
Shrimp dinner	10.0	n/a	457
Dairy Queen			
BBQ beef sandwich	4.0	1.0	225
Grilled chicken sandwich	8.0	2.0	300
Domino's			
10-inch pizza, 2 slices			
—ground beef	8.0	n/a	250
—mushroom and sausage	9.0	n/a	248
—pepperoni	10.0	n/a	265
—plain cheese	6.0	n/a	218
—sausage	8.0	n/a	246
14-inch pizza, 2 slices, plain cheese	7.0	n/a	281
16-inch pizza, 2 slices, plain cheese	10.0	n/a	478
Hardee's			
Hamburger	9.0	4.0	260
Regular roast beef	11.0	n/a	270

	TOTAL FAT (GRAMS)	SATURATED FAT (GRAMS)	CALORIES
Kentucky Fried Chicken			
BBQ flavored chicken sandwich	8.0	1.0	256
Long John Silver's			
Flavoredbaked foods:			
2-piece fish over rice, baked potato, green beans	10.0	n/a	518
2-piece fish over rice, side salad	9.0	n/a	345
1-piece chicken over rice, baked potato, green beans	8.0	n/a	448
1-piece chicken over rice, side salad	7.0	n/a	275
1-piece fish and chicken over rice, baked potato, green beans	10.0	n/a	538
Fish, 1 piece	3.0	n/a	90
Chicken, 1 piece	3.0	n/a	110
Seafood chowder with cod	6.0	n/a	140
Seafood gumbo with cod	8.0	n/a	120
Ocean chef salad	1.0	n/a	110
Creamy Italian dressing	3.0	n/a	30
McDonald's			
McGrilled chicken classic (plain)	3.0	n/a	250
Chunky chicken salad	5.0	1.0	160
Hamburger	9.0	3.0	270
Chef salad	11.0	4.0	210
McLean Deluxe	12.0	4.0	340
Taco Bell			
New Border Lites:			
Lite soft taco	5.0	n/a	181
Lite taco supreme	5.0	n/a	162
Lite soft taco supreme	5.0	n/a	199
Lite burrito supreme	8.0	n/a	350
Soft taco	11.0	n/a	223
Steak soft taco	9.0	n/a	217
Taco	11.0	n/a	180
Tostada	11.0	n/a	242
Chicken soft taco	10.0	n/a	223

	TOTAL FAT (GRAMS)	SATURATED FAT (GRAMS)	CALORIES
Wendy's			
Plain potato	0.0	0.0	310
Grilled chicken fillet	3.0	n/a	100
Caesar side salad	5.0	n/a	110
Sour cream and chive baked potato	6.0	n/a	380
Deluxe garden salad	6.0	n/a	110
Grilled chicken sandwich	7.0	n/a	290
Chili, small	6.0	3.0	190
Grilled chicken salad	8.0	n/a	200
Chili, large	9.0	n/a	290
Junior hamburger	9.0	n/a	270
Breaded chicken fillet	10.0	n/a	220
White Castle			
Fish sandwich without tartar sauce	5.0	n/a	155
Chicken sandwich	7.0	n/a	186
Hamburger	8.0	n/a	161
Cheeseburger	11.0	n/a	200
Side Orders			
Captain D's			
Rice	0.0	0.0	124
Baked potato	<1.0	0.0	277
White beans	<1.0	0.0	126
Corn on the cob	2.0	n/a	251
Green beans	2.0	n/a	46
Hardee's			
Mashed potatoes, 4 ounces	<1.0	0.0	70
French fries, small	10.0	n/a	240
Kentucky Fried Chicken			
Garden rice	1.0	0.0	75
Green beans	1.0	0.0	36
BBQ baked beans	2.0	1.0	132
Mean greens	2.0	1.0	52
Red beans and rice	3.0	1.0	114
Mashed potatoes and gravy	5.0	<1.0	109
Cole slaw	6.0	1.0	114

Fast Foods

	TOTAL FAT (GRAMS)	SATURATED FAT (GRAMS)	CALORIES
Kentucky Fried Chicken (cont'd)			
Macaroni and cheese	8.0	3.0	162
Potato wedges	9.0	3.0	192
Long John Silver's			
Green beans	<1.0	0.0	35
Baked potato	1.0	0.0	163
Rice	4.0	n/a	190
Corn cobbette	8.0	n/a	140
Cole slaw	6.0	n/a	140
Taco Bell			
Pintos and cheese with red sauce	9.0	4.0	190
Desserts			
Arby's			
Chocolate chip cookie (1)	4.0	n/a	130
Burger King			
Vanilla or chocolate shake	7.0	n/a	310
Captain D's			
Chocolate cake	10.0	n/a	303
Lemon pie	10.0	n/a	351
Dairy Queen			
Vanilla ice cream cone, small/regular	4.0/7.0	n/a	140/230
Chocolate ice cream cone, regular	7.0	n/a	230
Mr. Misty, regular	0.0	0.0	250
Yogurt cone, regular	<1.0	0.0	180
Yogurt cone, large	<1.0	0.0	260
Yogurt strawberry sundae, regular	<1.0	0.0	200
Chocolate sundae	7.0	n/a	300
McDonald's			
Soft-serve cone	<1.0	0.0	120
Strawberry sundae	1.0	0.0	240
Hot fudge sundae	5.0	n/a	290
Hot caramel sundae	3.0	n/a	310
Vanilla low-fat shake, small	5.0	n/a	310

	TOTAL FAT (GRAMS)	SATURATED FAT (GRAMS)	CALORIES
McDonald's (cont'd)			
Strawberry low-fat shake, small	5.0	n/a	340
Chocolate low-fat shake, small	6.0	n/a	350
McDonaldland cookies	9.0	n/a	260
Taco Bell			
Cinnamon twists	6.0	n/a	139
Wendy's			
Frosty, small	10.0	n/a	340

Resource 4
More Smart Choices

We gave you an example of a smart choice earlier. We recommended a McDonald's low-fat hot fudge sundae (only 5 grams of fat) instead of a Snickers bar with a whopping 14 grams of fat. Although you gain 10 calories, such a small gain is irrelevant because you are saving 9 grams of fat. This smart choice still provides a delicious chocolate treat. Below are more smart choices.

Note: Some products such as ice cream, yogurt, margarine, brownie mixes, and popcorn have a wide range of calories and fat grams. We used averages in the following comparisons.

		TOTAL FAT (GRAMS)	CALORIES
Not-so-smart	Snickers candy bar (2.07 ounces)	14.0	280
Smart	McDonald's low-fat hot fudge sundae	5.0	290
Savings		9.0	(+10)
Not-so-smart	Regular brownie mix (1 brownie)	9.0	190
Smart	Betty Crocker low-fat brownie mix (1 brownie)	2.5	130
Savings		6.5	60

		TOTAL FAT (GRAMS)	CALORIES
Not-so-smart	Regular margarine	11.0	100
Smart	Reduced-calorie/fat margarine	6.0	50
Savings		5.0	50
Not-so-smart	Tuna packed in oil (6¼-ounce can)	14.0	465
Smart	Tuna packed in water (6¼-ounce can)	1.0	186
Savings		13.0	279
Not-so-smart	Pudding with whole milk (½ cup)	5.0	100
Smart	Pudding made with skim milk	1.0	45
Savings		4.0	55
Not-so-smart	Jell-O instant sugar-free pudding: made with 2% milk (½ cup)	5.0	100
Smart	Jell-O instant sugar-free pudding: made with skim milk (½ cup)	1.0	90
Savings		4.0	10
Not-so-smart	One glazed yeast doughnut	25.0	465
Smart	Six slices toast with fruit spread	7.0	465
Savings		18.0	—
Not-so-smart	Regular ice cream (1 cup)	27.0	450
Smart	Healthy Choice low-fat ice cream (1 cup)	4.0	200
Savings		23.0	250
Not-so-smart	Frozen yogurt (1 cup)	6.0	250
Smart	Fat-free frozen yogurt (1 cup)*	0.0	205
Savings		6.0	45
Not-so-smart	Oil (½ cup)	964.0	108
Smart	Unsweetened applesauce (½ cup)**	53.0	<1
Savings		911.0	107

More Smart Choices

		TOTAL FAT (GRAMS)	CALORIES
Not-so-smart	Potato chips (1 ounce, about 6 chips)	11.0	160
Smart	Fat-free pretzels (1 ounce)	0.0	110
Savings		11.0	50
Not-so-smart	Potato chips (1 ounce, about 6 chips)	11.0	160
Smart	Mr. Phipps barbecue tater crisps (21)	4.0	130
Savings		7.0	30
Not-so-smart	Tostitos regular chips (1 ounce, 11 chips)	9.0	130
Smart	Tostitos baked chips (1 ounce, 13 chips)	1.0	110
Savings		8.0	20
Not-so-smart	Regular spaghetti sauce (½ cup)	6.0	140
Smart	Fat-free spaghetti sauce (½ cup)	0.0	80
Savings		6.0	60
Not-so-smart	Regular cheese stick (1)	5.0	70
Smart	Healthy Choice fat-free cheese stick (1)	0.0	45
Savings		5.0	25
Not-so-smart	Cottage cheese (½ cup, creamed)	5.0	117
Smart	Fat-free cottage cheese (½ cup)	0.0	70
Savings		5.0	47
Not-so-smart	Regular ricotta cheese (1 cup)	32.0	428
A little better	Part skim ricotta cheese (1 cup)	19.0	340
Really smart	Fat-free ricotta cheese (1 cup)	0.0	180
Savings (between regular and fat-free)		32.0	248
Not-so-smart	Microwave popcorn (3 cups)	7.0	130
Smart	Orville Redenbacher Smart-pop (3 cups)	1.0	50
Savings		6.0	80

		TOTAL FAT (GRAMS)	CALORIES
Not-so-smart	Egg (1)	5.0	75
Smart	Egg substitute (¼ cup)	0.0	30
Savings		5.0	45
Not-so-smart	Pecans (¼ cup)	18.0	187
Smart	Grape Nuts (¼ cup)	<1.0	101
Savings		17.0	86
Not-so-smart	Hamburger (6 ounces)	36.0	492
Smart	Bulgur (6 ounces)***	2.0	479
Savings		34.0	13
Not-so-smart	Dairy Queen Heath Blizzard	36.0	820
Smart	McDonald's low-fat shake	6.0	350
Savings		30.0	470
Not-so-smart	Otis Spunkmeyer chocolate chip muffin	28.0	500
Smart	Wheat bran muffin (recipe #33)	2.1	177
Savings		25.9	323

*Beware—there can be a tremendous difference in the amount of calories and fat among different brands of ice cream and frozen yogurt.

** Unsweetened applesauce can be substituted in equal quantities in recipes using oils. It works especially well in cakes and in fruit breads such as apple and banana.

***Bulgur (cracked wheat) is a good substitute for meat in chili, soups, and casseroles.

Part Three
On Your Own

Body Fat

Mini-Chapter 1

Survival of the Fattest

Only the strong survive. We all believe that, but is it true? Some experts believe that when it comes to humans, only the fat survive. Here's why.

In early evolutionary times, living was literally a feast or famine situation. If dad and his buddies were successful on the hunt, you feasted. If not, you had nothing to eat, and the famine lasted until the next successful kill. During times when food was scarce, people had to depend upon their own body's natural source of energy to get them through. They depended upon their stores of body fat, and those with the most fat had the best chance of surviving. This means, of course, that since those who store fat best survived, their genes were passed along to future generations.

Survivors were fortunate to have highly efficient fat cells that maximized storage capacity. Their fat cells were efficient because of a large supply of lipogenic enzymes whose purpose is to escort fat from the blood stream to the interior of fat cells. They also were fortunate to have a limited supply of lipolytic enzymes, whose purpose is to release fat from the fat cells so that it can be burned as fuel. These were advantages in the days of our early evolution when eating was unpredictable. Today they are a curse.

Today, we have cycles of crash dieting followed by binges. Ironically, the body responds very much the same way to these two extremes. When dieting, your body is thrust into a fat conservation mode. It perceives a famine, in other words, and tries desperately to protect existing fat stores to ensure survival. It does this by decreasing the supply of lipolytic (fat breakdown) enzymes. At the same time there is a diet-induced increase in lipogenic (fat buildup) enzymes, which causes your body to seize incoming fat and immediately store it. Your body does this even though it is desperate for fuel. The purpose of this ironic twist is to prepare fat cells to take advantage of any future feasts so that more fat than ever can be stored.

If fat is being protected during a crash diet, where does the body get its energy? Unfortunately, much of it comes from the muscles. While fat cells have protective enzyme systems to preserve fat stores, the muscles are vulnerable. Although the breakdown of muscles is devastating, the body views it as a positive occurrence when it is in a survival mode. This is because muscle is metabolically active, demanding a great deal of energy, and the less muscle you have the easier it is on the body to conserve energy.

When the diet is over, you of course gain the weight back quickly. You may not gain back all the muscle you lost, and probably won't unless you begin a vigorous exercise program. You will gain back the fat, however, and may gain back more than you lost owing to the zeal of your fat cells to store more than ever.

Every time you repeat a crash diet, things get worse. Your fat cells, having been through the diet wars a number of times, are now seasoned and have increased storage capabilities. This makes them more resistant than ever to relinquishing their fatty supplies. And the more resistant your fat cells become, the more vulnerable your muscles are to being torn down.

Now for the really bad news. The stricter the diet and the lower the caloric intake, the greater the damage. And the longer you continue the worse it gets. This means the most dedicated and iron-willed are penalized the most.

The bottom line is, you can't starve your fat cells. You must feed them and gently coax the fat out the Jack Sprat way, and this takes considerable time and patience.

Mini-Chapter 2

How Do You Wear Your Fat?

When you stand naked in front of a full-length mirror, what do you see? If you are a typical adult American you see an excess of fat peeking at you from various parts of the body. The exact location of that excess fat is important for two reasons. First, it may determine the degree of health risk associated with carrying excess body fat. Second, the location may dictate how easily that fat will come off.

When you wear a lot of fat around your waist, you take on the shape of an apple. This is called male pattern (also android, or abdominal pattern) obesity. Females tend to store fat on the hips, thighs, and buttocks, giving them more of a pear shape. This female pattern is also called gynoid, or gluteal-femoral pattern obesity. The apple shape is not necessarily restricted to men, although it is most prevalent in males. Similarly, the pear shape is not restricted to women.

Fat is stored in two primary ways—deep in the body cavities, and directly beneath the skin (called subcutaneous fat). Female pattern obesity emphasizes subcutaneous fat, resulting in jiggly thighs and unsympathetic comments from males. But most men have little room to boast and good reason to keep quiet: male pattern obesity emphasizes deep fat storage, which accumulates and pushes against the abdominal muscles, stretching them taut like a banjo string. This causes many men to incorrectly assume that because their protruding pot bellies are hard, they are not fat. This is a very wrong assumption and should be pointed out the next time an unwelcome comment surfaces about flabby female thighs.

Where fat is stored says a lot about how easily it can be burned off. Throughout the body, fat is stored in fat cells that comprise adipose tissue, a type of connective tissue. Dietary fat is stored in adipose cells with the aid of enzymes (lipogenic enzymes). Enzymes also play a role in calling fat from storage (lipolytic enzymes). Enzyme activity differs in various locations of the body, and this difference creates both good news and bad news.

The good news is, the lipolytic enzymes in the abdominal area are highly active and can call large amounts of abdominal fat out of storage and into the bloodstream. This means that given an appropriate low-fat diet and an increased regimen of daily physical activity, abdominal fat can be reduced rather efficiently. Though this is attractive from a fat loss perspective, it increases the risk of heart disease because when fat is dumped into the bloodstream in large amounts, it increases the body's production of cholesterol. But there's more to the story. Abdominal fat cells tend to be larger than those found elsewhere in the body, and these large fat cells are associated with glucose intolerance, increasing the release of insulin and the risk of maturity onset (Type II) diabetes. And since excess insulin can cause increased reabsorption of sodium by the kidneys, there may be an increase in blood pressure.

Fat stored on the hips, thighs, and buttocks also is a good news/bad news situation. The good news is, you can store a lot more fat below the waist (40-60 pounds) without greatly increasing the risk of heart disease. This is true for both men and women. The bad news is, the lipolytic enzymes that call fat out of storage are lazy in areas below the waist, and once fat is deposited in these areas, it's very difficult to remove.

The best way to determine your level of heart disease risk associated with fat storage is with the waist-to-hip ratio. Measure your waist without any clothing at the level of the navel to the nearest quarter of an inch. Next, measure your hips around the buttocks. Measuring the hips is a little tricky, so take several hip measurements, starting high on the hips and working down so as to get the largest measurement. Then divide the waist measurement by the hip measurement.

Hopefully, your hips are larger around than your waist. For women, a healthy goal is a ratio of approximately 0.80 or lower. A ratio of 0.80 is typical for young women, and increases progressively upward toward 0.90 by middle age. The ratio for men generally is not quite as good, because women have naturally broader hips. In young men, a typical ratio is approximately 0.90, and progresses with age to approximately 0.98.

The risk of heart disease is substantially higher in both sexes when the ratio reaches 1.0 and beyond. Although few women have such a bad ratio, the chances increase after menopause because abdominal fat storage increases more than lower body storage.

Mini-Chapter 3

Saddlebags and Love Handles

Fat that is deposited on the hips, thighs, and buttocks is zealously guarded by the female body. Fat in these areas is thought to have been deposited for a special purpose—providing life-saving nourishment for the newborn.

In times when food was scarce and unpredictable, Mother Nature had to be certain there would be adequate sustenance for new babies. She chose Mom's hips, thighs, and buttocks as storage sites, and she surrounded these areas with what at times seems like an impenetrable force field.

It is not uncommon for women to go to great lengths in an attempt to lose lower body fat. Some women take up marathon running, resulting in the loss of many pounds of body fat. Their faces become gaunt, their arms become pencil-thin, their waistlines shrink to less than 20 inches around. But despite all this effort, the fat on the thighs—the main reason for taking up running in the first place—is still pretty much intact. That darned force field.

So is it hopeless?

No. In most women, when they lose sufficient body fat, progressively more and more of it will come from the lower body. But not at first, and since most women do not stay on body fat reduction programs long enough to see the loss of lower body fat, they conclude that it's hopeless.

The Jack Sprat plan combined with moderate daily physical activity will eventually make an impact on the lower body fat of most women. We have seen successes, and Becca Coffin is an example. You must accept, however, that you may not progress to your desired goal—the slim, trim, 18-year-old cover-girl look—no matter how hard you try.

Failure to meet such an unrealistic goal is one reason that surgical liposuction techniques have become so popular. Liposuction is the "vacuuming out" of fat cells. It's a radical approach, but obviously one with lots of appeal, because plastic surgeons who perform liposuction are doing a land-office business. But bear in mind, this procedure is costly and not without risk. If too many fat cells are sucked out, for example, the area becomes concave, or sunken like a crater.

It's only fair to add that men seek out liposuction too. Their problem is love handles—those slabs of fat above the hips that hang over the belt. Like saddlebags (fatty deposits on the outer sides of women's thighs that give the thigh a shape like riding pants), love handles can bring tears to the eyes of even the most determined men. Why are love handles so stubborn? We know it's not because the fat there is being protected to provide energy to a newborn. Why then? No one is certain. But love handles appear to be an early site of fat deposition, and it's possible that the body employs a "first in/last out" scheme.

In addition to liposuction, a variety of quick-fix schemes have popped up. You should be aware of them in order to protect yourself from being taken in.

Thigh Cream

It was just a small scholarly study of 11 women reported to a professional group, the North American Association for the Study of Obesity, at an annual meeting. But it set off a storm of consumer interest when researchers reported recently that a cream made from a common asthma medication (aminophylline) seemed to slim women's thighs and to flatten the ripples of cellulite.

For five weeks, several women applied the magic cream to one thigh and massaged it in. An inactive cream was applied to the opposite thigh. The treated thigh was reported to shrink a full one and one-half inches!

Is there anything to this? Or is it just a lot of foolishness that will soon bilk female consumers out of their hard-earned cash?

At first glance, it seems like a story right out of the tabloids. Various bogus creams have been sold over the years, with claims that they remove cellulite or increase breast size. Could this asthma cream be different? Maybe, but it's a long shot.

Perhaps the cream's active ingredient, when rubbed on the thighs, stimulates those lazy enzymes we described earlier. And once stimulated, the enzymes help move fat out of the adipose tissue and into the circulation.

If this is possible (and as yet, it's much too early to tell), it is important to point out that the cream does not cause the fat to disappear. It merely makes the fat available to be burned off. You still have to expend the effort to burn the calories.

There is also the possibility that there is no basis to this claim. The researchers did not measure the fat content of the thigh. Instead, they depended on circumference measurements. Such measurements are notoriously difficult to reproduce accurately, and even a slight displacement up or down could add or subtract volume substantially.

There is no doubt we will be hearing a lot more about this. In fact, during the months we spent writing this book, a number of companies have stepped forward and are marketing thigh cream. As yet, however, no real evidence has been produced to support a positive effect—other than a positive effect on the economy.

Postpartum Window of Opportunity

Recent research suggests that during breast-feeding after pregnancy, fat deposits on the hips, thighs, and buttocks are vulnerable to reduction. The factors that guard this fat are temporarily removed, and fat from these areas can be more easily mobilized and used as fuel to support the newborn. Unfortunately, this opportunity arises when Mom has more important things on her mind than exercising or eating smarter to reduce the size of her thighs. Mom has to concentrate on being Mom, and in so doing, she misses the brief window of opportunity that has been opened to her.

Six months to a year after childbirth, Mom gets the urge to get back in shape. But by then, her body may be undergoing change again, back to her former state. But all is not lost. It just might take a little longer.

We are aware that losing lower body fat can be frustrating and can cause you to take foolish steps. One such step is the purchase of costly creams and lotions. The other is investment in fancy exercise equipment that guarantees fat loss in specific areas. Sorry. Such quick fixes don't work.

Mini-Chapter 4

Cellulite

Cellulite. Say the word, and images of waffled thighs and rippled butts appear. Say the word, and drive women to tears, then to the drugstore in search of the latest lotions and potions. Billions have been spent in the vain attempt to rid ourselves of this fiend. Jack Sprat estimates that he could have been a very wealthy man if it wasn't for all the money his wives squandered on gimmicks to rid themselves of dreaded cellulite.

Why would the Creator curse us with such a mean-spirited and persistent foe?

She didn't. So-called cellulite is no different from other fat deposits. It's just plain old fat that looks different. Here's why.

Your body stores fat in crescent-shaped connective tissue cells called fat cells. Fat cells have a tremendous storage capacity, and when they are full, they look like blown-up hot-water bottles.

If we could peek beneath the skin at a fat pad, we would see a crisscrossing matrix of connective-tissue strands that form compartments similar to those of a beehive. When the fat cells that fill each compartment expand, the compartments swell, pressing against each other and forcing an outward bulge that pushes toward the skin. When this occurs, several factors will determine whether you develop the unsightly waffled look.

Women are more susceptible to the cellulite look than men because women store more of their fat just beneath the skin, whereas men store more of their fat as deep fat in the abdominal cavity. The more fat you have just beneath the skin, the more likely bulges will show.

Even when men have a large stockpile of fat beneath the skin, they will often escape the rippled look. This is because the outer layers of women's skin may be thinner than those of men, showing the contents underneath more clearly. Also, the connective tissue compartments (of the beehive) may be tighter and more restrictive in women, and that increases the tendency of fat cells to bulge outward to a greater degree.

The effects of these collective factors are exaggerated in women because women concentrate their fat storage in the hips, thighs, and buttocks. If fat stores were more evenly distributed around the body, the bulging, rippled effect would be reduced substantially.

The concept of cellulite being a "different animal" was promoted by women's magazines and those who wanted to sell salves, creams, and other bogus items to help get rid of this problem. Cellulite looks different, and because it shows up on the hips, thighs, and buttocks, it's very difficult to get rid of. But cellulite is not different from fat elsewhere on your body, and it doesn't require special interventions. The Jack Sprat plan is all you need.

Mini-Chapter 5

Snakes and Snails
and Puppy Dog Tails

Until puberty, little boys and girls are pretty similar in body composition. With puberty, the hormones take over, and girls add fat, boys add muscle. The "typical" young adult female body is about 20 to 25 percent fat, 37 percent muscle, 14 percent bone, and 25 percent organs.

The proportions in a "typical" young adult male body are somewhat different, with 15 to 18 percent fat, 45 percent muscle, 15 percent bone, and 25 percent organs.

In both sexes, "essential" fat is stored in the marrow of bones, throughout the central nervous system, and in the heart, lungs, liver, and other major organs. This fat, which makes up approximately 3 percent of total body mass, plays an important role in the functioning of your body.

Women have additional essential fat that is tied to childbearing and the "fleshing out" of the female figure. This accounts for 5 to 9 percent more essential fat. This means that the leanest female will be in the neighborhood of 8 to 12 percent fat, whereas males can reduce all the way to 3 percent fat. It's possible if there is a great excess of muscle present, for the essential fat of males to be an even lower percentage.

Beyond the essential fat is storage fat. In days when food was scarce, stored fat pulled us through. Today, with fast-food restaurants on every corner, fat storage has skyrocketed. It's typical, starting at age 21, to add about 1 to 2 pounds of fat per year to the storage pool. A combination of factors brings this about.

For the first 21 years of our lives, we eat food that will sustain an active lifestyle in a body that is growing and developing.

Then, in our twenties, growth and development stalls, we find *real* jobs, get married, have babies, and do all sorts of things, except be physically active. In addition, year by year, our basal metabolic rate declines, causing us to burn off progressively fewer calories.

The weight we gain is seasonal, typically from Thanksgiving through the New Year. Then, when the weather warms and the days lengthen, we lose much of what we gained. But not all. There generally is a residual of about one pound that stays with us and accumulates year by year. This is called creeping obesity, and it progresses well into middle age before our body weight tends to level off.

Unfortunately, the fact that our weight levels off does not mean the process has ceased. Weight levels off because you start losing muscle, which balances fat gain. This means you get fatter without it necessarily showing up on the bathroom scale.

Mini-Chapter 6

Pinch an Inch

Americans are too fat. We all know that. But just how fat are we?

That's harder to say than you might think. Stepping on a scale is helpful, but it can be confusing because your weight tells you very little about how fat you are. National Football League players who weigh well over 200 pounds, most of which is muscle, show how misleading judging fatness by weight can be. And most popular height/weight charts provide such wide ranges of acceptable weights that experts question their usefulness.

So what's the answer?

Muscle is more dense than water, whereas fat is less dense. Muscle sinks, fat floats. For a quickie test on your own, do a turtle float in the swimming pool. As you float, blow out all the air in your lungs. Do you continue to float, or do you sink like a rock? If you float, or if you only sink a little bit, guess what? That's right. Fat city.

A variety of body fat measurement methods have been developed over the years. The most accurate way is the hydrostatic (underwater) weighing technique. Unfortunately, it is time-consuming, awkward, requires sophisticated equipment and technical know-how, and usually is only available in university exercise physiology labs.

There are easier and quicker methods available that take measurements of subcutaneous fat—the fat stored directly under the skin. Such methods assume that subcutaneous fat makes up a particular proportion (usually about 50 percent) of total body fat. The other 50 percent is stored deep in the body, in and around the liver, heart, and other organs, in bone marrow, and so forth. It's true that approximately half the body's fat is located under the skin in young adults, but the exact amount can vary tremendously. What's more, with age, the distribution of fat changes and a greater proportion is stored internally.

This means, if the way your body stores fat does not agree with the general assumptions made regarding fat distribution, the number you get from an easier fat assessment method can be way off the mark.

The best of the easier methods is the fatfold, or skinfold —"pinch-an-inch"—test. Subcutaneous fat is measured at several body sites by grasping the fat under the skin and pulling it away from the underlying muscle. The thickness of the fold at several points in the body is measured with spring-loaded calipers that close on the fold. The measurements are used in a formula that tries to predict what body fat would be if the hydrostatic weighing procedure were used.

A variety of high-tech methods—bioelectrical impedance, ultrasound, fiber optic probes—are used in health clubs to try to estimate the quantity of subcutaneous fat. In the bioelectrical impedance method, muscle offers less resistance than fat to the low-level electrical current that is passed through the body. This is because muscle contains a greater concentration of water and electrolytes (salt, potassium, and the like). The resistance encountered reflects the amount of fat present. At least that's the way the system is supposed to work. Unfortunately, chances are good that you will get a bogus reading with the bioelectrical impedance and other high-tech methods. And if you do, you won't know it, because you have nothing to compare it to.

We offer this advice. Because life is too complicated as it is, and because high-tech hocus-pocus methods (which promise simple answers to complex questions) are likely to disappoint, you are better off just to take your clothes off and stand in front of a full-length mirror. A good long look will tell you everything you need to know about body fatness, and probably more than you want to know. But it's necessary. And as you progress on the Jack Sprat plan, use the mirror to reflect your improvement.

Mini-Chapter 7

Don't Sweat It

Since the Roman Empire, people have assumed that sitting in oppressive heat is good for you. There is not much evidence to support this notion, but health clubs and manufacturers of saunas and steam baths do all they can to keep the idea alive. They claim, for example, that profuse sweating provides a deep cleansing of the skin that is otherwise impossible to attain. They claim that the limp noodle feeling you get from an extended stay in the heat is the ultimate in relaxation. And, of course, because the pounds literally melt off, a stint in the heat is touted as the ideal way to control weight.

The problem is, of course, that a fat body isn't suffering from an excess accumulation of water. The hurtful comments from your mother-in-law are not about the water that has accumulated around your waist, or on your hips, thighs, and buttocks.

Although we can't lose fat by sweating, we sure can lose a lot of water. It's no problem to sweat off one quart per hour sitting in the sauna: that's a two-pound weight loss (one pint of sweat weighs one pound). Do a little exercise while in the sauna, and you can double sweat loss to about 4 pounds an hour.

Shrinking Cells

Losing water weight makes you feel slimmer. You're not, of course. Here's how it works.

Losing water from the body results in dehydration, an unhealthy condition your body cannot tolerate for long. At first, you lose water from just beneath the skin, from the interstitial fluid outside the cells of your body. As the interstitial fluid level drops, fluid is coaxed from inside the cells to sustain fluid balance inside and outside. This causes the cells to shrink, and explains how water loss can lead to lost inches.

As more fluid is lost from the body, water is transferred from the bloodstream to balance the continued loss of interstitial fluid. Now you're in trouble. A low water level in the blood means a decreased blood volume. This puts pressure on the heart to circulate the blood at a faster rate, because there is less of it. In addition, there is an imbalance of electrolytes—salt and potassium—which can cause the electrical system of the heart to go haywire. Other problems surface as well, but you get the idea. Dehydration is nothing to play around with.

Fortunately, your body is smart enough to correct the situation as quickly as possible by holding on to all the liquid it can. Soon, the pounds you lost in the sauna are right back on. All that was accomplished was putting your health in danger, especially if you have any preexisting conditions, such as high blood pressure or heart disease.

Fat Loss in the Sauna?

The latest flimflam scam involves telling people they will lose fat in the sauna. When you evaporate sweat, energy is required (to convert a liquid to a gas). If you evaporate a lot of sweat, you use a lot of energy, and you lose fat. Sounds good. But it doesn't work.

The explanation is rather technical, but it can be boiled down to this: The energy that is used to evaporate sweat from your skin comes from the heat provided by the sauna, not from within your body. Since your body isn't supplying the energy, you don't burn off any fat.

A Word of Caution

With all that said, are we advising you never to go into a sauna? Not at all. Use it to unwind, if you like, but not as a means to lose weight. Just keep the following in mind to ensure safe use:

- Increase your fluid intake to replace fluids lost as sweat. A 1-pound weight loss means you are a pint low on body fluids.

- Stay away from alcohol and caffeine. They accelerate fluid loss from the body.
- If you are taking any medication, or if you have any preexisting medical conditions, be sure to check with your doctor to make certain that you aren't putting yourself at risk.
- Keep your sessions relatively short.

Mini-Chapter 8

Baby Fat

Body fat is stored in crescent-shaped cells called fat cells, which make up adipose tissue (a type of connective tissue). A hot time for fat cell development in the body is during the third trimester of pregnancy and the first two years of life. The more the mother eats and the fatter she becomes, the greater the number of fat cells developed in the fetus. And if the parents subscribe to the thinking that a fat baby is a healthy baby, millions more fat cells are added over and above the generous number that will be created naturally. This overabundance of fat cells can aid fat storage later in life and create a lifelong weight management nightmare.

Sensitive to this dilemma, many parents took off in the opposite direction, bent on raising lean and mean offspring. Skim milk was used, as well as other low-fat foods. Taken to the extreme, however, this well-intended strategy backfired. Newborns are in a dynamic state of growth, and dietary fat and cholesterol are vital to development. Studies have reported that babies deprived of adequate dietary fat and cholesterol demonstrate retarded development.

But don't interpret this as meaning it's best to pack on the pork. Moderation is the key. Don't eat for two when you're pregnant, and don't try to mold your offspring after the Pillsbury Doughboy. Eat sensibly while pregnant and gain weight in accordance with your physician's directions. Gaining more may add additional unwanted fat cells to the developing fetus, while gaining less could cause development problems. The same is true with the newborn.

As a rule of thumb, do not worry about restricting fat and

cholesterol intake for the first two to three years of life. Mother's milk will take care of nutrient needs, of course. But for those not breast-feeding, follow standard medically prescribed formulas. After your child reaches age three, you can cut back gradually on fat intake. Not only will this not cause a problem, but starting at such an early age could help your youngster avoid obesity later on.

TV's Fat Kids

A recent study by researchers at the Center for Science in the Public Interest should prod every parent into action. They monitored five TV stations in the Washington, D.C., area on Saturday morning and found that 60 percent of all commercials were for food, and 96 percent of these commercials were for fatty fast foods, chips of all kinds, candy, sugary cereals, salty canned foods, and the like. Of the 222 commercials observed, just one mentioned eating more fruit and grains. And even that recommendation was in the context of eating a not-so-ideal cereal.

These commercials have a huge impact on food choices. The influence of TV runs deep and may last a lifetime, especially when combined with watching Mom and Dad consume grown-up versions of the Saturday morning fare.

Is there anything you can do? A hard-liner would tell you to turn off the TV, or even get rid of it. But that would be too severe, and the resulting chaos would beat parents into submission quickly. Besides, Mom and Dad like to watch TV too.

You might start by gradually reducing TV watching from an average of seven or more hours per day to two hours on weekdays and perhaps an extra hour or two on weekends. This will prevent your children from vegetating in front of the set and will force everyone to make choices based on quality of viewing. Experts suggest that children can respond positively to this restriction if you approach it as a family decision and allow everyone a voice.

But what about Saturday morning, when damaging commercials peak? How can you modify the damage without interfering with this most sacred of tiny-tot times? And, more important, how can you do this without forcing Mom or Dad to climb out of bed hours before they intend to?

Try this. Use a VCR to record the cartoons and let the kids watch them at another time. Encourage the kids to zing through the commercials just the way Mom and Dad do.

I'm sure there are lots of other ways to attack this problem that are more creative than ours. Use your best judgment, but whatever you do, do something.

Diet and Exercise

It's frustrating for parents of overweight kids because they know what their kids will face as they get older. The jokes, the stigma, the discrimination. We are frequently asked to provide a diet and exercise program to help kids reduce. No problem. As far as diet is concerned, your kids will eat what you eat. So get started cleaning up your diet, and the kids' eating habits will surely follow.

As far as exercise is concerned, the answer is simple too. Turn off the TV. Kids don't need a special exercise program. They are, in fact, amazingly creative at inventing clever physically demanding games if given the opportunity. But the opportunity does not arise when sitting transfixed in front of the TV set.

To test this out, try turning off the TV on a rainy afternoon when the kids are stuck in the house. Their energy level will drive you nuts, as they bounce of the walls and dash up and down the halls. All you have to do is encourage this release of energy for an hour or more each day, and that will be plenty of exercise.

Mini-Chapter 9

Fat, Hormones, and Breast Cancer

Can a low-fat diet help prevent breast cancer? Many experts say no. Others say, emphatically, yes. The confusion stems partly from how low-fat a low-fat diet must be to have an impact.

An oft-cited 1987 study showed that a 30 percent fat diet did not significantly lower the incidence of breast cancer. One interpretation is that this proves that a low-fat diet is of no benefit. A better explanation is that because a 30 percent fat diet is not a low-fat diet, you wouldn't expect it to have much of an effect.

Despite the fact that the American Cancer Society and the American Heart Association recommend a 30 percent fat diet, the preponderance of evidence favors a much lower guideline of no more than 20 percent fat. (Remember what we told you in chapter 5.) Unfortunately, a truly low-fat diet is often not used in scientific studies, in favor of the American Heart Association's fatty diet.

So where is the evidence linking dietary fat and breast cancer? The evidence has been available for more than a decade, but it has been poorly distributed. The first major breakthrough was a comparison of the incidence of breast cancer among Japanese versus American women. Breast cancer in Japan is rare, whereas in this country breast cancer is common, attacking more than 10 percent of all women.

This comparison was initially dismissed as meaningless because it's possible that cultural differences were operating. In other words, Japanese women have a natural immunity.

Not so. When Japanese women move to the United States and eat like Americans, their incidence of breast cancer skyrockets. The difference is the 15 percent fat diet of those in Japan compared with the 37-40 percent fat diet of Americans. Similar results have been observed repeatedly when comparing vegetarians and nonvegetarians within the same country.

If dietary fat is at least partly responsible for breast cancer, how does it work?

Some people think the problem is the storing of fat in the breasts, creating fatty tumors. It is likely that the process is more complicated with a number of possible mechanisms. A diet high in fat, for example, causes increased production and increased biological activity of estradiol, the main estrogen. This in turn may encourage the development of breast tumors.

There is evidence that the immune system is weakened by a high-fat diet. This is a potentially critical factor because the immune system provides our first line of defense against the initial attack of cancer and against the spread of cancer if it gains a foothold.

An indirect effect of high-fat diets also may be operating. High-fat diets composed of meat and dairy products are low in fiber, and fiber helps trap and remove estrogen in the digestive tract. A low-fiber diet would be ineffective in removing estrogen from the system.

Here's another possible explanation. The risk of breast cancer has been linked to early puberty. In countries where fat is scarce, puberty is delayed to the age of 15 to 19, and breast cancer is rare. In the United States, puberty is common in girls 11 to 13 years of age, and the incidence of breast cancer is high.

Whatever the exact mechanism behind breast cancer, it would appear that consuming a diet high in fat helps it along. Moreover, it seems reasonable that a low-fat diet would go a long way toward helping to prevent breast cancer and some other forms of cancer, as well (such as colon and prostate cancer). In fact, estimates from the National Cancer Institute indicate that possibly 80 percent of cancers could be prevented by stopping smoking and switching to a low-fat diet.

We have made great progress as a society in quitting smoking. Now it's time to do the same with dietary fat. Unfortunately, there's a big fly in the ointment. It wasn't difficult for us to accept the fact that smoking is bad for our health. But it's a little tougher to convince ourselves that such sacred cows (no pun intended) as whole milk, cheese, hamburgers, meat loaf, hot dogs, bologna, salami, steaks, and fried chicken are bad for our health. But we'll keep trying, and who knows? Maybe someday we'll get through to the masses.

Mini-Chapter 10

Miracle Fat Pills

As long as obesity is a problem, there will be flimflam schemes to get rid of it. And with our society's dependence on medications, there's no doubt that new pills will continually be manufactured as "magic bullets" designed to make us slender and beautiful forevermore.

The latest entrant into the "magic bullet" arena is a pill that allows 30 percent of the fat eaten to pass through the body undigested. This means that if you take in 100 grams of fat, only 70 will be digested, which has the effect of lowering the fat content of a 2,400-calorie diet from approximately 37.5 percent to 26 percent. Since each gram of fat equals 9 calories, not digesting the 30 grams (30 x 9 = 270 calories) would reduce caloric intake by 270 calories. Over one year's time, this would add up to (all things being equal) a loss of 28 pounds of body fat.

How does it work?

It inhibits an intestinal enzyme (pancreatic lipase) that helps digest fat. Because fat molecules are too large to be absorbed through the walls of the intestines, they must be broken down, and pancreatic lipase helps get the job done. But, if fat is not broken down, because there are not enough enzymes around, it passes through undigested.

Research studies show dramatic weight loss among patients taking the enzyme pills. But hold on before you get too excited.

First of all, the drug is still in the early experimental stage and probably will not be eligible for FDA approval for years. And when it is, it most likely will be a prescription drug intended for the obese patient—not for losing 10 pounds prior to your twenty-year high school reunion.

Second, and more important, is the question of long-term benefits. It's not hard to produce big results in the short run—ask anyone who has crash dieted, lost a lot of weight, then gained it all back and more. The long-term implications are the most important, and the long-term implications of the enzyme pill are unknown. We do know, from research on other artificial "quick and easy" methods of weight loss, that once the weight loss procedure is discontinued, the weight comes back with a vengeance. The reason is, patients haven't learned to eat a healthy low-fat diet and have depended totally on the artificial treatment.

Researchers for new drugs like to point out that part of the therapy accompanying the drug should be training people to follow a low-fat diet. If this is the case, why bother giving the drug in the first place? Why not simply begin eating in a healthy low-fat way that will gradually cause a reduction in body fat. And once you reach your body-weight goal, you will have mastered correct eating habits that will sustain your new body weight for the rest of your life.

In contrast, taking drugs will accelerate the weight loss process, but no lasting benefit is accrued. On the contrary, the drugs probably will create a psychological and/or physiological dependence, and once the drug is discontinued, the "crutch" is removed, resulting in a deep sense of abandonment. Old dieting habits are picked up again, and because the body's metabolism is in a state of disarray, the weight comes back quickly.

Unfortunately, the powers-that-be believe it is impossible for the masses to change their lifestyle. Part of this, of course, lies in the fact that there is no profit associated with a change in lifestyle, whereas there is tremendous profit in selling drugs. In addition, many experts in the medical community believe the masses need medication to help lose weight, because being too fat is a disease just like high blood pressure and should be treated similarly. As long as this thinking prevails, we will continue to indulge in expensive and potentially health-destroying drug-induced yo-yo dieting.

Admittedly, there may be certain types of obesity that are caused by a chemical imbalance. The same may be true for various psychoses and/or criminal behavior, and in such cases, treatment can and probably should take a medical course similar to treating hypertension. But should the masses who truly have the capacity to change their lifestyle, and who have the capacity to be captains of their own ship, sell out for a pill? The answer is no. But they probably will, given the persuasive powers of multi-million-dollar advertising.

Fat Gene

Will discovery of the "fat gene" lead to drugs that will truly offer long-term help to the more than one-third of Americans with weight problems?

Don't hold your breath.

Discovery of the so-called fat gene may not be as significant as the hype would have us believe. That doesn't mean it's not an important discovery. On the contrary, it may be a major breakthrough in genetic research. The problem is, it may offer little relief to the overweight masses.

The gene in question is thought to secrete proteins that control satiety—a sense of satisfaction that you have consumed enough food. If you have inherited the "correct" gene, signals from the gene are sent to the hypothalamus (part of the brain that controls appetite) telling it that you have had enough to eat. The "fat gene" doesn't send this signal, and (it is assumed) you just keep right on eating. The solution, then, is to supply a drug that does the job of the faulty gene, and BINGO!—no more overeating, and no more weight problem.

While this sounds good—scientific and all—it depends entirely on the assumption that obesity is an organic problem. Something is wrong with the body's physiology, in other words. This is certainly true in some cases. Hypothyroidism (underactive thyroid) is one example. But this is a tiny portion of the total population of obese individuals, and most obesity experts would reject the organic explanation as entirely too simplistic. Indeed, the causes of obesity and contributions to it are many.

People often eat for emotional reasons, and the more emotionally involved they are (bored, depressed, excited, what have you), the more they eat. This is true regardless of appetite. People in our society regularly engage in "automatic eating"—eating in which you are essentially unconscious of what and how much you are consuming because your attention is directed elsewhere, perhaps toward watching TV. The organic explanation also discounts the impact of food choices. Eating dietary fat makes you fat, whereas eating carbohydrates and proteins will assist you in managing your weight. This is true even if you are consuming the same number of calories of each. And, don't forget physical activity. It is well documented that the obese are much less active compared to those of normal weight in our society.

If you are overweight, it's entirely possible that you don't have the faulty gene but are guilty of emotional eating, automatic eating, eating too much fat, and/or being too inactive. If so, taking drugs to correct a faulty gene would be of no benefit.

Mini-Chapter II

Brown Fat versus White Fat

There are two types of fatty tissue found in the body. When you pinch an inch from your midriff or thigh, you are pinching so called white fat. This is overwhelmingly the most prevalent type of fat in the body, comprising about 99 percent. The remaining fat is called brown fat and is located in small amounts around the neck and on the back and chest.

Brown fat differs from white fat because it has a high rate of metabolism, whereas white fat is practically metabolically inert. When brown fat "turns on," it can burn an extraordinary number of calories that are used to generate heat. Brown fat can be turned on after a large meal or during exposure to cold. The latter is the case for animals that hibernate: they tend to have large stores of brown fat.

Years ago when brown fat was first discovered, some scientists speculated that differences in the amount of brown fat may determine who gains body fat and who doesn't. A person with hefty portions of brown fat would be expected to be leaner, in other words, than one with smaller brown fat stores. When it was later determined that the amount of brown fat was minuscule, this line of reasoning was dismissed.

Despite the small amount of brown fat on the human body, there is renewed interest in its potential to combat obesity. Recent research suggests that even a very small amount of brown fat could account for a meaningful portion of the resting energy expended in humans. If this is true, it could be a major player in avoiding obesity. Let's take a look.

The average adult woman between the ages of 30 and 60 and

who weighs about 135 pounds would have a basal metabolic rate of about 1,300 calories (kcals) per day. This is the amount of energy expended per day at rest that is required to keep the body alive and well. (Energy expended in work and physical activity would be added to this for an overall daily energy expenditure.) If the energy expended at rest could be increased by, say, 10 percent for an hour or two after meals, this would increase overall daily energy expenditure by 20 calories or so.

Although this doesn't sound like much, over one year's time this adds up to 7,300 calories, or the equivalent of about 2 pounds of body fat. Since most Americans gain weight gradually at the rate of approximately 1 to 2 pounds per year from young adulthood through middle age, the impact of brown fat to raise metabolic rate slightly could potentially reverse this trend.

At the present time, scientist are trying to determine whether brown fat truly plays a role in the development of obesity, or if it's another example of a theoretical concept that doesn't pan out in the real world.

Healthy Eating

Mini-Chapter 12

Counting Calories Can Be Misleading

Counting calories can be misleading, especially when it comes to judging the potential impact of a low-fat high-carbohydrate diet. This is because the body is very efficient at storing dietary fat as body fat and very inefficient at converting carbohydrate to body fat. Here's an example.

Let's assume you take in 2,000 calories a day and that 40 percent of those calories are in the form of fat. This means that you are taking in 800 calories of fat per day. If you burned off half of those fat calories in your daily activities, that would leave you with 400 calories to store. To convert dietary fat to body fat requires a 3 percent tariff, or 12 calories of the 400. This means that 388 calories of dietary fat (a little more than one-tenth of a pound) would be stored as body fat.

Let's assume that you begin a low-fat high-carbohydrate diet, but you still consume 2,000 calories per day. Let's assume that all other things are equal, but instead of confronting 400 excess calories of fat, you confront 400 excess calories of carbohydrate. Since your body doesn't like to convert carbohydrate to body fat, it would first try to store it as glycogen (strings of glucose molecules). If that didn't work, it would be forced to convert the excess carbs to fat. To convert carbohydrate to body fat requires a whopping 23 percent tariff. So 92 calories of energy would be used of the 400 calories available, leaving only 308 for storage.

The difference in these two scenarios—308 calories stored as body fat versus 388—is substantial and could mean the difference of 5 pounds of stored body fat over six months. And when you add in the efforts the body makes so as not to be forced to convert carbohydrates to fat in the first place (storing carbs as glycogen), you can see that simply counting calories can be very misleading when judging the benefits of a low-fat high-carbohydrate diet.

Mini-Chapter 13

The Lowdown on Sugar

Up to this point most of our fury has been directed against dietary fat, and for good reason. Sugar can be destructive, too, but before we get into that, let's clear up some confusion about what exactly sugar is.

Simple carbohydrates are usually referred to as sugar. There are two types: monosaccharides and disaccharides. Among the monosaccharides are glucose (also called dextrose), fructose (fruit sugar), and galactose. Disaccharides contain combinations of two monosaccharides. Sucrose (table sugar), for example, contains glucose plus fructose, and lactose (milk sugar) is glucose plus galactose. You get the idea.

Simple carbs can be bad guys but not as bad as once thought. In the past, sugar was blamed for just about every ailment, including obesity. We now know that dietary fat—not sugar—is the primary cause of weight gain. If combined with dietary fat, however, sugar helps the body store fat more efficiently. The problem is that simple carbs are digested rapidly, rushing into your bloodstream, causing an outpouring of insulin in response to the onslaught of sugar. It's the insulin that helps store dietary fat as body fat. The best way to gain body fat, then, is to have a soft drink with your burger, or to pour sugary ketchup on your fries.

The quick digestion of simple carbs also causes wide shifts in blood sugar, which can affect how you feel throughout the day. A midafternoon candy bar might give you a quick pickup (because of the rush of blood sugar), but it's soon followed by a major letdown because the big insulin response causes your blood sugar level to plummet. This can leave you hypoglycemic and feeling worse than before.

Simple carbs cause tooth decay. That's well established, and it's a good reason to cut back. Sugary products also often provide only "hollow" calories—with little or no nutrients. We call these junk foods. Eating too much junk food can be a health problem, especially for the elderly, who tend to eat less and might be filling up on sugar and avoiding the things they should be eating.

Complex carbs, in contrast, are good guys. They are commonly called starch. Examples are potatoes and other veggies, pasta, oatmeal, and bread. Starch, of course, wasn't always seen in a positive light, and crash dieters once were warned to avoid starch at all costs. Unfortunately, avoiding starch is a primary reason their diet resulted in the loss of muscle and water instead of body fat. It's also the primary reason the diet failed.

Complex carbs are formed when three or more glucose molecules combine into a polysaccharide. Complex carbs take longer to digest than simple carbs, and the sugar enters the bloodstream more gradually, which prevents a major outpouring of insulin. This has a stabilizing effect on blood sugar concentration. That's why a midafternoon complex carb treat (a whole wheat muffin, for example) will gradually pick you up and keep you up.

Complex carbs are loaded with nutrients, and they tend to be bulky, which makes it difficult to overconsume on calories. In fact, a great way to lose weight is to eat lots of complex carbs every day. You will be consuming plenty of food and feel satisfied, yet the pounds will melt off.

Another type of complex carb is fiber. It is resistant to digestive enzymes, causing it to leave a residue in the digestive tract. Fiber is an important component of a healthy diet.

With this as background, you can see that when we refer to sugar in lay terms, we are actually referring to monosaccharides and disaccharides—or simple carbs. And when we refer to complex carbs (starch), we are actually referring to polysaccharides.

The Scoop on Sugar

In this country, as much as half of our carbohydrate intake, and 25 percent of our total daily calories is in the form of sugar. That equates to about 120 pounds a year. Most of us are unaware that we eat this much sugar, because we don't pile it on at the dinner table. Unfortunately, sugar is a leading additive (along with salt and fat) in processed foods, and our diet is heavily loaded with processed foods.

Surprisingly, you can avoid "sweets" and still get megadoses of sugar from foods that don't taste sweet, like soups, salad dressing, condiments, cereals, and canned and frozen foods, including canned and frozen vegetables. You also can get simple sugar naturally from fruit, molasses, honey, maple syrup, and the like. Still, only about one pound in four of the sugar we eat comes from natural sources. Fruit is a good choice because it contains fructose. Although fructose is a monosaccharide, it is digested slowly, which dampens the insulin response. Fruit and molasses are good sources of sugar, because they provide nutrients along with the sugar.

Honey is an excellent natural source of sugar—about 40 percent of which is fructose. But claims that honey contains valuable potassium, iron, calcium, and such tend to be overblown. The amounts are extremely small and probably inconsequential.

How much sugar should we eat?

Because we can get all the monosaccharides we need from complex carbs, technically, we don't need to eat any sugar. Experts suggest that we dramatically reduce our intake of sugar to no more than 10 percent of total calories. That's about 10 to 15 teaspoons of sugar per day, depending on how many calories you normally consume.

Unfortunately, it's hard to tell how much sugar you are getting in your diet. Food labels aren't much help because they may list sugar under a variety of names, including barley malt or concentrated fruit juice. New labeling laws are supposed to correct this by combining all sugars, regardless of type, under one heading. Whether this will be sufficient to provide consumers with accurate information remains to be seen.

Is eating sweets an acquired trait? No. Infants like sweets. But how much we prefer is learned. Growing up on sugary cereals (with extra teaspoons of sugar on top), soft drinks, ice cream, and candy teaches us to enjoy highly sweetened foods. Can this be reversed? Of course. Like anything else, take it one step at a time. Start with something easy, like tea or coffee. Simply quit putting sugar in it. At first it will taste funny, but eventually it will taste normal to you. And when sugar is added, it will taste too sweet. It's possible to retrain your taste buds. All it takes is a little determination.

Mini-Chapter 14

Protein

Americans have had a sustained love affair with protein. It's the darling of the dietary world; it can do no wrong. When you were a kid, Mom and Dad might have let eating your veggies slide, but there's no way you were going to skip out without eating your meat and drinking your milk. Why? Because they are the all-important protein foods, that's why.

Fortunately, as the luster has worn off meat and fatty dairy products and we see them for what they really are, so too has the luster begun to fade on protein. Protein is now being viewed in its true light, as a double-edged sword. One edge builds strong bones and muscles. But the other edge, the edge that cuts us deeply, arises from the way protein comes to us—wrapped up in a blanket of fat, and saturated fat in particular.

To prove this point, consider the five leading sources of fat in the American diet: (1) ground beef products (hamburgers, cheeseburgers, meat loaf); (2) processed meats (luncheon meats, hot dogs); (3) whole milk and whole milk products, including cheese; (4) doughnuts and other baked goods; (5) beef steaks and roasts.

What is most prevalent on the top-five list? The answer is, protein foods. Foods our parents revered as healthful. Foods we were taught to hold sacred. Nearly every adult grew up believing he or she should drink at least three glasses of whole milk every day, and most Americans eat meat at least twice daily.

We were raised to think of these foods as protein foods. But what are they, really? In truth, they are fatty foods that also happen to be rich in protein. We all would be much better off if we switched our attention to plant protein as our primary source. Unfortunately, at present we get by far most of our protein from meat, dairy products and eggs, and only a small portion from rich plant sources such as beans and grains.

But what if you switch to a low-fat diet? Does it matter whether you still eat meat and dairy products? Apparently, yes. Studies have shown that when people switched from a meat-based low-fat diet to a plant-based low-fat diet (with soybeans as the major source of protein), blood cholesterol concentration dropped by 25 percent.

Why should it matter whether you eat meat or not as your source of protein, as long as you are on a low-fat diet? The reason, researchers believe, is that plant proteins such as soy have a unique pattern of amino acids that help lower cholesterol.

The fact that protein generally comes wrapped in fat is a problem. But it's not the only problem. Protein itself in large amounts can be destructive to the body. A good example is osteoporosis—wasting of the bones. With age, the bones lose calcium and become fragile. Loss of calcium is owing to several factors, including lack of exercise, hormonal changes, and probably aging itself. Another key player is protein intake. When you eat a lot of protein, the by-products of protein metabolism can bind with calcium, which gets lost in the urine. Thus, a case can be made for decreasing protein intake, while increasing calcium intake, as an effective way of fighting osteoporosis.

Because osteoporosis is caused by the loss of calcium from the body, the dairy industry advocates its products as a means of getting more dietary calcium and thus helping the bones stay healthy. Sounds logical, doesn't it? It is, but too much emphasis on dairy products can push protein intake to high levels, causing an increased loss of calcium from the body, which can make the problem worse.

The by-products of protein digestion also can place undue stress on the kidneys, especially as the years roll by, possibly accelerating aging of these important organs. This is because large amounts of water are needed to accomplish the considerable waste removal associated with protein digestion. It is well established that people with kidney disease do much better when their protein intake is reduced substantially, sparing their weakened kidneys from having to work so hard to process all those by-products. Excess protein also can increase risks of dehydration, especially in people who exercise heavily or who work in hot environments. And the liver is victimized by a high protein intake, too, because it is the liver that must metabolize protein at the expense of considerable energy and resources.

Are we saying that everyone should avoid protein?

Of course not. Protein is a critical component of a healthy diet. It not only helps build strong bones and muscles, it bolsters the immune system, keeps the nervous system intact, aids wound healing, contributes to healthy skin and hair, aids the digestive process by helping the body break down and absorb nutrients . . . you get the idea. But just because protein is important to us, doesn't mean that "more is better." On the contrary, more can be harmful.

When the RDA for protein was established years ago, there was concern that people were not getting sufficient protein in their diets. Protein was harder to come by then, and there was the need to emphasize its importance. One way to do this was to set a high RDA, so high that if you failed to achieve it, even by a fairly wide margin, you would still be getting sufficient protein. Today, not only do most of us achieve the RDA, we far exceed it. The average young adult American probably consumes one-and-one-half to two times the RDA for protein. Young males are likely to consume as much as 120 or more grams of protein per day, even though they require less than 60 grams.

The bottom line is, you need protein in your diet, but not as much as you may think. Watch your intake and try to slant it toward plant sources as much as possible. Your body will thank you.

Mini-Chapter 15

Fake Fat and Fake Sugar

We have finally realized that dietary fat is a bad hombre, and we're doing something about it. To be sure, we haven't made many healthful changes in our diet. That would be asking too much. But we have plunked down big dollars for "fake fat" items, providing, of course, that there is little if any sacrifice in taste. What are these fake fats?

There are a number of fat replacement products on the market and certainly more to come. The current batch are made from egg proteins, milk, and a variety of carbohydrates that are heated, reduced to their basic components, and blended with water to resemble fat and to reproduce, at least partially, the taste of fat. Although there is less taste, there also are fewer calories than in real fat, and fake fat doesn't clog the arteries.

Fat substitutes that have been around for a while include polydextrose and maltodextrin. Polydextrose is used in frozen desserts, puddings, and cake frostings. It contains only 1 calorie per gram, compared with 9 calories per gram for fat. Maltodextrin contains 4 calories per gram and is used in margarines and salad dressings.

There is a new class of fat substitutes that seems to reproduce the creaminess of fat more effectively than the two above. Simplesse is a processed protein created by heating and blending egg whites (or milk) until they evaporate into misty particles. This creates a sense of creaminess, which is missing in polydextrose and maltodextrin. Simplesse is used only in cold products such as ice cream, yogurt, dips, salad dressings, and mayonnaise because it loses its creamy texture when heated.

Olestra is a synthetic combination of sucrose polyester and fatty acids. It contains fat, but because of the way it is formulated, the body cannot digest it or absorb it, and therefore it doesn't contain any calories. Olestra can be used in the same way as natural fat, and without restriction. It can be heated and used as cooking oil, or cooled and used in ice cream. Olestra is not available to the public, but look for FDA approval in the near future.

Will fake fat help us win the battle of the bulge? It's hard to predict. But a note of caution is in order. Many of the fat-free products are loaded with sugar, especially the baked goods. Although sugar is not quite as bad for you as fat, it's not that far behind. And eating too much excess sugar can put pounds on too.

Speaking of sugar, when artificial sweeteners were introduced, we thought we had the magic bullet. You could drink soft drinks all day long and not gain an ounce. But it didn't turn out that way, and obesity in this country is at an all-time high. The reason is unclear, but it may be that people "added" products with artificial sweeteners to their diet instead of "substituting." It also has been suggested that sweeteners do not fully satisfy our craving for sweets. If not, we charge into our lunches or dinners hungrier than we thought, and we tend to overindulge.

Mini-Chapter 16

The Lost Fiber of Our Society

Fiber is the Rodney Dangerfield of the American diet. It gets no respect. But it should. Without adequate fiber our gastrointestinal (GI) tract suffers greatly. Fiber provides roughage that helps foodstuff move along, and smoother and quicker movement means fewer GI problems. Fiber also helps in the battle against obesity. It affords no calories and provides, because of its bulk, a feeling of fullness and satiety. Caloric absorption from other foods may decrease as well, possibly by as much as 3 percent (that's 60 free calories in a 2,000-calorie per day diet).

But Americans don't take advantage of the gifts fiber brings to the table. We ought to consume at least 20 to 35 grams per day. Instead, the average American gets considerably less than this amount. This is owing to our heavy dependence on meat and dairy products and our reduced consumption of vegetables and fruits. Our compulsion to process foods is also to blame. The milling of whole grains cuts the fiber content at least in half, which allows the flours to bake into lighter fluffier goods but robs the digestive system of a valuable commodity.

There are two types of fiber: soluble and insoluble. The type discussed above is insoluble and is found in the skins of fruits and vegetables, in grain products such as wheat bran, and in whole-grain cereals and bread. It gives bulk to the stools and softens them, acting as a natural laxative and reducing the likelihood of swollen rectal veins—a.k.a. hemorrhoids. The laxative effect also helps prevent bulging of the bowel into pockets (diverticulosis) which can become infected (diverticulitis) to the point of requiring surgery. More serious problems can be avoided with fiber too. Research suggests that cancerous activity in the colon may be triggered by waste products allowed to remain in prolonged contact with bowel walls. Sufficient fiber moves things along, keeping exposure time to a minimum.

There's more good news when it comes to fiber. The other type—soluble fiber—is called soluble because it dissolves in water. Its claim to fame is that it helps reduce serum cholesterol. Here's how it works.

In the intestines, soluble fiber forms a gel that coats the walls and prevents reabsorption of bile (the yellowish green liquid manufactured in the liver and stored in the gall bladder that helps break down ingested fat). The body normally likes to reuse bile, releasing it, reabsorbing it back into the gall bladder, then releasing it again. This recycling system is highly efficient, and only a small amount of bile gets lost each time it is released.

When bile is lost, more must be produced. And since cholesterol is the principle raw material used to make bile, the need for new bile persuades the body to pull cholesterol out of the bloodstream. This results in a lower cholesterol level. Although the reduction may amount to only a 3 to 10 percent drop, when combined with a low saturated fat diet, the overall effect can be substantial.

Good sources of soluble fiber include oat bran, rice bran, and some cereals. Check the labels carefully to make certain you are getting a hefty dose of fiber.

A word of caution. Fiber foods can be gas-producing and can cause gastrointestinal discomfort, especially if your system isn't used to getting sufficient fiber. Be patient. Your body will adapt as your intestinal chemistry needs time to get used to the change. If you find the discomfort too intense, however, cut back and build up gradually. Your goal is at least 30 grams a day. Is this a lot? Yes, compared with what the typical American takes in. But, no, when considering that residents of Third World countries consume more than twice this amount, and rural Africans may consume over 100 grams per day. In such cultures, problems we take for granted—constipation, hemorrhoids, appendicitis, diverticulitis, and colon cancer—are virtually nonexistent.

Mini-Chapter 17

Vegetarianism

The definition of a "vegetarian" has changed quite a bit in recent years. At one time, only people who avoided all foods of animal origin were considered vegetarians. Today, we call these folks vegans (vee-ghans). There are several other types of vegetarians, defined by what foods of animal origin they eat.

Lacto-vegetarians eat dairy products. Ovo-vegetarians eat eggs. Lacto-ovo-vegetarians eat dairy products and eggs. Pesco-vegetarians eat fish, dairy products, and eggs. Semi-vegetarians eat dairy products, eggs, and a little fish and chicken. Some who include occasional red meat in their diet also consider themselves semi-vegetarians.

The Jack Sprat diet could be characterized as semi-vegetarian. Although we firmly believe that a vegetarian diet (which may include some fish, a little skim milk, and so forth) is best, we realize that such a diet may represent too great a change initially for the masses. As such, if you follow the Jack Sprat diet, you will find that you are eating red meat, chicken, and such, but only occasionally. And when you feel comfortable with this, you may decide to take things a step further.

A recent survey found that 12 million Americans claim to be vegetarians. This is a substantial increase in the ranks, but because of the variety of types of vegetarians and the looser definitions, it is difficult to compare these results with earlier surveys. In the past, most people who became vegetarians did so for ethical, religious, or environmental reasons. Nowadays many are joining the ranks to improve their health. Vegetarians generally have little problem with weight management. They eat and eat all day long, but consume relatively few calories because the foods they eat are not calorically dense. This is because they are low in fat. What's more, the risks of chronic diseases such as heart disease, stroke, diabetes, and several forms of cancer (breast, prostate, colon) are much reduced among vegetarians.

That's not to say that all vegetarian diets are healthful. If you eat fatty dairy products—especially whole milk and cheese—and egg yolks, you may consume as much fat and saturated fat as red-meat-eaters.

An issue that always arises when discussing vegetarianism is getting adequate dietary protein. Vegetarian diets can easily supply all the protein you need. In fact, most of us probably consume as much as two times the amount of protein our bodies require. At issue is the challenge of getting "complete" protein—protein that contains all the essential amino acids. (Essential amino acids are those that your body cannot manufacture and that must be obtained from the diet.) Foods of animal origin contain all the essential amino acids. Nonanimal foods contain some, but not all, and for this reason it is necessary to combine foods. Red beans plus rice is an example of each food providing what the other lacks.

Combining foods is not as difficult or as inconvenient as you might think. For one thing, you don't have to combine foods within the same meal as was once thought. You do, however, have to get all of the essential amino acids throughout the day.

If you decide to go all the way and become a vegan, it's best that you educate yourself with a "how-to" book to make certain you are considering all of the issues. For example, some vitamins and minerals are not easy to get if you avoid animal products. Examples include vitamins B-2 (riboflavin), B-12, and D, and the minerals calcium, iron, and zinc.

Vitamin B-12 is the one meat-eaters always point to as a reason not to quit eating red meat. They have a point. Most experts agree that B-12 is found only in foods of animal origin. Others suggest that some plants may contain B-12, but this is controversial. Vitamin B-12 deficiency is rare in this country, because we eat huge quantities of red meat and dairy products. If you don't get enough B-12, anemia (weak blood) may result. Other problems include swelling and cracking of the tongue, hypersensitive skin, and peripheral nerve degeneration.

Surprisingly, research shows that vegans usually have normal vitamin B-12 status. How is that possible if they shun red meat and dairy products? They don't even eat fish and shellfish, which contain a modest amount of B-12. This is a puzzle. Perhaps vitamin B-12 is gotten from fortified nutritional yeast, or B-12 fortified soymilk. Many vegans take brewer's yeast, baker's yeast, or live yeast, but some experts claim that you aren't likely to get sufficient B-12 from these sources. Perhaps they are getting their B-12 from other fortified foods and supplements. Regardless, the fact remains that not receiving B-12 from animal sources can be overcome.

Calcium is the mineral pointed to by nonvegetarians as problematic. It is critical to your health, especially to the prevention of osteoporosis (wasting of the bones). The main source of calcium in the American diet is milk and milk products. But if you give up milk, you will have to get your calcium from vegetables. Fortunately, you can get calcium from broccoli, blackstrap molasses, brussels sprouts, chickpeas, collards, figs, great northern beans, kale, kidney beans, mustard greens, navy beans, okra, pinto beans, prunes, rhubarb, soybeans, spinach, and turnip greens. And if you still eat seafood, you can get calcium from oysters, salmon, sardines, scallops, and shrimp.

A word of caution. Although the American Dietetic Association says vegetarianism is suitable for children, make certain that nothing essential is left out of the diet. The same is true for pregnant or breast-feeding women, the elderly, and those with debilitating diseases. If there is a question, seek professional advice from a dietitian or nutritionist.

Mini-Chapter 18

Antioxidants

Supplements—to take or not to take? We spend billions of dollars each year on vitamins, minerals, and all sorts of supplements ranging from garlic to bee pollen. Some people buy them because their doctor recommended them; others operate on their own. To most of us, supplements represent a form of nutritional insurance. If we miss out on certain vitamins or trace minerals, pills will meet the need.

Most of us believe at least some of the foolishness that is tied to the marketing of supplements. Most believe, for example, that extra vitamins provide more pep and energy. Unfortunately, some people get sucked into the supplement lifestyle, and their lives revolve around a never-ending series of pills, potions, and powders.

What's the truth?

It's hard to say. Talk to a professional dietitian or nutritionist, and you will likely hear that you don't need supplements if you regularly consume a well-balanced diet. There are exceptions, of course. People who don't easily absorb naturally occurring vitamins or minerals may need a boost. The elderly often need supplements because their appetite wanes, and they simply don't get enough of what they need.

In general, professionals support the notion that there isn't a strong scientific basis for taking supplements. This means, for example, that scientists haven't been able to prove that taking extra vitamin C helps prevent the common cold, or that vitamin E prevents heart disease. But this argument can work both ways. Scientists haven't been able to prove conclusively that vitamin C does not prevent the common cold. This is because proving or disproving something like this takes lots of research, supported by lots of dollars, over a number of years.

The ability of vitamins to neutralize free radicals is one promising area of research that has received a great deal of publicity. Free radicals are produced by the body constantly as an offshoot of metabolism. They're bad dudes that can wreak damage throughout the body. They can, for example, oxidize materials—such as fat—found in muscle cell membranes. They erode your muscles, in other words, and are believed to be tied into the aging process.

Enter the antioxidants. Vitamins C and E and beta carotene are touted as effective antioxidants that prevent free radicals from doing their thing. Several research studies have reported good results from taking extra amounts of these antioxidants. For example, one study found that because metabolism increases during exercise, free radicals increase too. Runners who consumed large daily doses of vitamin C (1,000 mg), vitamin E (600 IU), and beta carotene (50,000 IU) produced one-third fewer free radicals during an exhausting 35-minute run.

Such results are interesting but hardly conclusive. In the meantime, it's up to you to determine whether antioxidants and other supplements are worthwhile. You must decide whether or not to shell out the extra bucks for a bottle of pills. As far as cost is concerned, it's hard to determine whether one product is better than another. Is an organic vitamin C pill better than one built in the lab? There is no conclusive proof one way or the other, but a good argument can be made on the organic side.

What about dosage? Will megadoses make you safe, or sorry?

Moderation is generally best. But for argument's sake, let's take a look at the recommendations of Dr. Linus Pauling. His views on vitamin C are so controversial that he has been called a kook.

Kook, indeed! Dr. Pauling's research in physics and chemistry is widely respected. He is known as the father of molecular biology and molecular medicine. He has won the Nobel Prize, not once but twice, in 1954 and in 1962 for work unrelated to vitamin C.

Dr. Pauling is known for advocating megadoses of vitamin C to prevent the common cold. His supporters cite studies in which vitamin C in doses of at least 1 gram (1,000 mg) and often as much as 3 grams a day succeeded in preventing colds. (In comparison, an 8-ounce serving of orange juice provides 120 mg of vitamin C.)

Studies also are cited in which doses of vitamin C were helpful even after the cold had struck. The cold was milder, the course shorter. Recent research suggests that super-high doses of vitamin C (more than 3 grams a day) may help in fighting cancer and even AIDS.

Scientists generally don't accept that megadoses are useful, however. This is because not all research results on vitamin C are positive; plus there is some question as to the safety of taking such high doses. Those who oppose taking megadoses point to potential toxic problems, including the formation of kidney stones, upset of the body's acid-base balance, and the destruction of vitamin B-12.

Although these effects are possible, research hasn't seen them arise with daily intakes as high as 3 grams. Some bad effects have been observed at doses of 3 grams and lower, however, including nausea, abdominal cramps, and diarrhea. Expectant mothers are warned to keep vitamin C intake in check because of potential negative influences on the fetus.

The controversy is heated in part because of the extreme positions involved. The establishment insists that the body's need for vitamin C is small: the recommended daily allowance is only 60 mg, the amount needed to prevent scurvy.

What does Dr. Pauling recommend?

He has determined that the body needs about 12 grams (12,000 mg) of vitamin C each day—the equivalent of 100 glasses of orange juice. He bases this amount on the observation that most animals manufacture their own vitamin C internally, and they make (relative to their size) about 12 grams a day. Only a few species, including humans and other primates, lack the capacity to produce vitamin C, so they need an outside source.

Is Dr. Pauling correct? Who knows? Perhaps we'll have answers in the near future. The recent interest in vitamin C as a potential protective measure in the fight against heart disease has spurred researchers to take a closer look.

Free radicals may be involved in atherosclerosis (clogging of the arteries). Since clogged arteries are the underlying cause of 95 percent of all heart attacks, the intake of antioxidants may be very important as a preventive health measure. A recent scientific study spanning ten years revealed that men who took extra vitamin C were 42 percent less likely to die of any cause, and 45 percent less likely to die of cardiovascular disease when compared with men who consumed relatively little vitamin C. Similar results were found in women too.

This raises the question, how much "extra" vitamin C was taken by the healthier group? A health-enhancing effect wasn't found until the daily vitamin C intake was increased to about 200 mg a day. Thus, it seems reasonable to suggest that taking extra vitamin C, in the range of 200 mg to 12,000 mg (according to Dr. Pauling), may improve health. Exactly how much is needed remains to be determined, however.

What about garlic and other more exotic supplements?

Again, the jury is still out. Garlic began receiving attention as a healthful agent several years ago when it was discovered that the incidence of heart disease was substantially less in Mediterranean countries compared with the United States.

Although many factors could be responsible for this, including a slower pace of life, less stress, and less meat and dairy product consumption, researchers seized upon the high intake of garlic as a factor. Since then, studies have suggested that garlic may help reduce LDL-cholesterol (the bad kind that leads to clogging of the arteries), increase HDL-cholesterol (the good kind that helps prevent clogging), and reduce the stickiness of blood (the tendency of blood to clot).

But before you rush out and purchase garlic pills, consider the following. The subjects in these studies ingested a large amount of garlic, the equivalent of 10 cloves a day. That's a lot, and most people would find it unpleasant to eat that much. Moreover, most people would experience side effects like diarrhea, nausea, and vomiting, not to mention the body odor and horrible breath that accompany garlic consumption.

Because of the need for ingesting large amounts, manufacturers introduced garlic pills. This solved one problem but created another. The processing required to reduce garlic to a pill may destroy the biologically active and healthful compounds. Manufacturers are aware of this problem, and most advertise that their product retains its potency. Is this true? Your guess is as good as ours.

The bottom line is there may be something quite good about taking extra doses of some vitamins, minerals, and other exotic supplements. The problem is separating fact from fiction. Unfortunately, reliable scientific evidence is very slow in coming. And because those who sell these agents stand to make a profit from your purchase, they are not dependable sources of information. So, it looks as if you are on your own. Read and learn as much as you can; then make your choices. Good luck.

Mini-Chapter 19

New Food Labels

The food labels now required by the Food and Drug Administration are an improvement over the old, but they certainly are not nearly as useful as they could be, especially when it comes to helping consumers trim fat from their diet. The new labels still don't, for example, tell you what percentage of calories are in the form of fat. As you can see on the "reduced fat" peanut butter label shown here, near the top you get total calories per serving and fat calories, but no percentage.

Nutrition Facts			
Serv. Size 2 Tbsp (36g)		Servings 14	
Calories 190		**Fat Cal** 110	
Amount/Serving	%DV*	Amount/Serving	%DV
Total Fat 13g	**20%**	**Total Carb** 12g	**4%**
Sat Fat 2.5g	**13%**	Fiber 1g	**8%**
Cholest 0mg	**0%**	Sugars 3g	
Sodium 170mg	**7%**	**Protein** 9g	**11%**
Vitamin A 0% • Vitamin C 0%			
Calcium 0% • Iron 4% • Niacin 25%			
Vitamin B6 6% • Folic Acid 6%			
Magnesium 15% • Zinc 6% • Copper 10%			

*Percent Daily Values (DV) are based on a 2,000 Calorie Diet

To compute the percentage of fat, you have to divide the fat calories (110) by the total calories per serving (190) and multiply by 100. When you do, you find that the "reduced fat" peanut butter is 58 percent fat. Hardly a low-fat item, and knowing that it's 58 percent fat helps you to quickly arrive at that conclusion.

But how many consumers will take the time to do the calculations required to determine the percent fat? The answer is, not many. Instead, most will glance a bit further down the label to where it says "Total Fat, 13 grams, 20%." And they will make the mistaken assumption that this 58 percent fat product is only 20 percent fat.

What does the 20% on the new label mean if it doesn't stand for the percentage of fat per serving? It means a serving represents 20% of the total daily allowance (or daily value) of fat.

Pretty confusing, huh?

Needlessly so, unfortunately. Here's how it works.

The new labels allow 65 grams of fat per 2,000 calories per day. This amount of fat represents 30 percent of total daily calories. From the label above, you can see that a serving contains 13 grams of fat, which is 20 percent of the daily allotment of 65 grams—thus the 20% on the label. Most people are surprised and chagrined to learn that a product they thought was 20 percent fat is actually 58 percent.

Obviously, there are several problems with this new labeling scheme.

First, few people carry around in their heads a menu of everything they are going to eat in a day. This makes the fat percentage that is reported virtually meaningless to those who are sufficiently well informed to know what it's supposed to represent.

Second, the fat content guideline is much too high. A 30 percent fat diet is a fatty diet that will make you fat and will contribute to heart disease, diabetes, and various forms of cancer. Unfortunately, because the new labeling system has chosen to use a 30 percent fat guideline, the masses will incorrectly assume that a 30 percent fat diet is healthy.

Finally, the guideline for saturated fat is much too high, allowing 10 percent of total calories. The body does not require any saturated fat, and saturated fat does only nasty things once it invades your system. A healthful guideline is cut your saturated fat intake to as close to zero as possible.

Are there any positive aspects of the new labeling system when it comes to dietary fat? Yes, but not many. In the past, you were not told how many calories of fat were contained in a serving. You used to have to multiply the number of grams of fat times 9 to find out. Now you don't have to do that. In the old system, saturated fat content was not prominently stated, and often absent. Now it's obvious.

Why don't the new labels offer more help to struggling consumers? That's hard to say, but some things are clear. Those who truly have the health of our nation at heart (no pun intended) were either excluded from the process or ignored. Another possible factor is powerful business interests. Most decisions made in this country are compromises that land somewhere between what's best for us and what's best for business profits. Many powerful businesses would suffer severe cuts in profits if Americans began to eat a healthier low-fat diet. Could such businesses have influenced the process of choosing a new labeling scheme, knowing that a confusing and misleading scheme is almost as good as not having a new scheme? Who knows? But keep in mind that business interests were able to delay substantially introduction of the new Eating Right Pyramid (which replaced the old unhealthy four food group concept), because of its emphasis on low-fat foods.

Here's some advice regarding how to cope with the new labels. First, forget the percentages. If they don't confuse you, they will mislead you. Second, count fat grams and allow yourself no more than 45 grams per 2,000 calories: that's a little more than 2 grams of fat per 100 calories, and it represents a healthy 20 percent fat diet. Third, beware of saturated fat and avoid products containing more than 1 gram per serving.

Mini-Chapter 20

If You Booze, You Won't Lose

A drink here and there probably won't hurt, but a couple of drinks a day can add up to lots of extra pounds. The reason is, although alcoholic beverages are fat-free, they are very high in calories with 7.1 calories per gram and 201 calories per ounce. At that rate, it's easy for the total calories to mount up. Let's take a look.

Twelve ounces of light beer can have 80 to 130 calories, and 12 ounces of regular beer averages about 146 calories. A 3.5 ounce glass of wine can vary from 70 to 80 calories for dry wine to up to 150 calories for a sweet dessert wine. A 3-ounce daiquiri has about 122 calories, a 3.5-ounce martini about 140.

One of the main problems with alcoholic drinks is their hidden presence. Most people don't consider them as dietary items, and most are surprised to learn they are fattening. Over the years we have interviewed many people who cannot understand why they are having so much trouble managing their weight. With analysis we usually find the problem is the predinner martini, dinner wine, and a late-night nip. This is not considered excessive, and many might view it as typical. Typical or not, it adds 300 to 500 useless calories per day, and the body cannot cope with a constant deluge of additional calories without adding body fat.

But the alcohol story has an interesting twist. The calories from alcohol tend to add more fat to men than women. The reason is, women tend to be smarter about managing their total caloric intake, especially when it includes alcohol. They recognize alcohol's caloric value and tend to exchange alcohol for other high energy goods, generally sweet things. Men, on the other hand, simply add alcohol to their diet.

There's another interesting twist. So called social drinkers (no more than two drinks per day) are more likely to get fat than heavy drinkers. This is because heavy drinkers tend to concentrate on drinking while neglecting their eating. But don't heavy drinkers take in a lot of calories each day in the form of booze? Yes, they do. But the effect is much different from consuming those calories in the form of food. The reason is, excessive alcohol intake interferes with the digestion and absorption of other foods, which reduces the total calories available to the body. In addition, alcohol engages in some rather peculiar metabolic interactions in the body, which may cause it to burn faster and less efficiently when taken in large amounts.

These effects help to keep weight down. Unfortunately, they also reduce the availability of important nutrients, possibly leading to malnutrition. This explains why an alcoholic may not be obese despite consuming more calories than a nondrinker.

There are two additional points of concern for women to consider. First, men and women may handle the effects of alcohol differently. Researchers have found that when men and women consume an equivalent amount of alcohol (based on their body weight), the blood alcohol of women remained higher than men's. This may be owing to a lessened ability of women to begin breaking alcohol down in the stomach. Thus, a given amount of alcohol will affect a woman more strongly; she will "feel" it faster, and it may impair her abilities to a greater extent. All in all, this may help to explain why, all things being equal, drinking alcohol may have a more damaging effect on a woman's body than a man's.

Second, alcohol may contribute to premenstrual syndrome (PMS). Experts suggest that PMS sufferers cut back on alcohol consumption, especially during the days immediately prior to each menstrual period.

Mini-Chapter 21

Salt

Americans eat way too much salt. Salt is so plentiful, in fact, that there is no RDA (recommended daily allowance), because there is no worry about a shortage of it in the diet.

Salt is actually a compound of sodium and chloride, and it is the sodium content in salt that is worrisome. In fact, when we talk about salt, we are actually talking about the sodium in salt. To avoid confusion, you must understand that about 40 percent of salt is sodium. One teaspoon equals about 5 grams of salt, containing approximately 2 grams of sodium. The typical American consumes about 6 to 18 grams of salt per day, or about 2.4 to 7.2 grams of sodium.

You can monitor either your daily salt or your daily sodium intake. Monitoring sodium is probably easier because it is listed as sodium on labels. Our bodies require only a fraction of the amount usually consumed, no more than about 1 gram of sodium daily.

Why is salt so bad for you?

Years ago, it was assumed that if you ate too much salt your blood pressure would go up, and if you cut back on salt your blood pressure would drop. The latest research suggests a more complicated relationship, but it still supports cutting salt intake as a way to reduce blood pressure. Even a drop in blood pressure of only 2.5 points (millimeters of mercury) could reduce the death rate from heart attacks by 5 percent and from stroke by 9 percent. The effects of cutting back on salt are greater in those over 50.

But cutting salt intake is not easy, because you first have to find it. The latest research suggests that we get only about 6 percent of our salt from the salt shaker, and only about 5 percent from salting while cooking. This means that our major source of salt intake is hidden. Canned foods, and soups in particular, are notoriously high in sodium. Other foods to avoid: cheeses; foods prepared in brine, such as pickles and sauerkraut; processed meats, especially luncheon meats; salty fish; snacks commonly made with salt added, such as potato chips, pretzels, popcorn, and peanuts; bouillon cubes; seasoned salts; sauces such as Worcestershire, soy, and barbecue; and condiments such as mustard, ketchup, and horseradish.

Read labels, and you will find large amounts of sodium in unexpected places. A serving of cornflakes, for example, contains more sodium than a serving of cocktail peanuts. The peanuts taste saltier because the salt is on the surface and provides a concentrated dose.

Watch out for compound words that include the word sodium. For example, MSG, monosodium glutamate, is a form of salt, as are sodium bicarbonate and disodium phosphate.

Mini-Chapter 22

Does Dietary Cholesterol Matter?

The day we discovered that a high concentration of cholesterol in the blood causes heart attacks was the day dietary cholesterol became a pariah—something to be avoided at all costs. Food manufacturers began putting large red labels on their products proclaiming proudly, "NO CHOLESTEROL!" Mothers who care for the health of their families gobbled up the red-labeled products while cutting back on shrimp and eggs and everything else they could think of that contained hefty amounts of cholesterol.

What did this flurry of activity accomplish? A major reduction in the nation's blood cholesterol levels?

Sorry, but the effect was much less than hoped for. The reason is, we failed to understand the relationship between dietary cholesterol and the cholesterol that circulates in the blood. When you eat cholesterol, it doesn't necessarily raise the concentration of cholesterol in your blood. And when you cut back on dietary cholesterol, your blood cholesterol concentration does not necessarily drop. This is because the vast majority of cholesterol in your blood is produced within your body, primarily in the liver, and saturated fat is the raw material used in the process. When you eat cholesterol, production of cholesterol in the liver shuts down momentarily to compensate for the incoming supply. Then production picks up again. This means, the blood concentration of cholesterol stays more or less the same.

The story changes, however, when you ingest saturated fat. The more saturated fat you eat, the greater the cholesterol production in your liver and the greater your blood cholesterol concentration. So, if you want to take a swipe at your blood-cholesterol level, cut your saturated fat intake.

Ironically, many of the red-labeled "no cholesterol" foods are loaded with saturated fat. And though we give these products to our families for the purpose of lowering their blood cholesterol level, in actuality we are contributing to a higher level.

So, what's the word on shrimp and other high-cholesterol foods? Can you eat as much as you'd like?

No. Moderation is the key, and it's best to keep your dietary cholesterol intake down to about 200 mg a day. There are two reasons for this. First it's possible that if you load up on dietary cholesterol, eating huge amounts day after day, you may overwhelm your body and the mechanisms that control cholesterol production in the liver, and the result could be a boost in your blood cholesterol level. Second, most foods high in cholesterol also are high in saturated fat. Take the egg, for example. For years, eggs have been viewed as a bad guy because of the high concentration of cholesterol—about 212 mg per yolk. And while Americans have been avoiding eggs as a means of lowering their consumption of cholesterol, they unwittingly also have been rewarded with a reduction in saturated fat intake. Avoiding meat and fatty dairy products also causes a reduction in both dietary cholesterol and saturated fat.

In fairness to the egg, it should be pointed out that egg whites are a wonderful food that is high in protein and nutrients, while virtually devoid of cholesterol and fat. Throughout the Jack Sprat diet, when a recipe calls for an egg, we substitute two egg whites. Same effect as far as taste is concerned, but much healthier.

There is another matter to consider when it comes to dietary cholesterol and heart disease. Even though dietary cholesterol seems to have little effect on the blood cholesterol concentration, it appears nonetheless to contribute to heart disease.

How? No one seems to know. It has been suggested that people who consume high amounts of cholesterol also consume high amounts of saturated fat, and it is actually the saturated fat that is doing the damage. But even when the saturated fat factor is taken into consideration, the relationship between dietary cholesterol and heart disease stands.

The bottom line is, keep your dietary cholesterol intake to a minimum. Although a lower intake of dietary cholesterol may not lead to a lower concentration of cholesterol in the blood, it will contribute to a lessened overall risk of heart disease. If you follow the Jack Sprat diet, your intake of cholesterol will be reduced to healthful levels. The same is true for saturated fat.

Mini-Chapter 23

Phytochemicals

The latest rage in the world of nutrition is phytochemicals
—from the Greek *phyto,* which means plant. These substances,
which until recently were unknown, are believed to protect
plants from harmful sunlight. They may do more than that for
humans, and some experts are suggesting they may be the best
friend we've ever had, because they may block key steps in the
development of malignant cancer cells. And you can bet that if
any of the scientific claims about phytochemicals hold water
through the rigorous testing that's sure to come, you will soon
see bottles of phytochemical pills shoving aside vitamins and
minerals on the shelves of your local drug store.

Until now, we believed that, because vitamins and minerals
promote health and prevent disease, the most important thing
was consuming adequate quantities of each, regardless of the
source. Though this still may be true, a good argument is brew-
ing that you can't take the vitamins and minerals separate from
the food source and expect to get the full effect. The discovery of
the potency of phytochemicals, in other words, raises the specter
that broccoli is healthful not only because of its vitamin and
mineral content but because of its phytochemicals. And as such,
taking vitamins and minerals (known to be contained in broccoli) from a bottle may produce little of the healthful outcomes
associated with eating the broccoli itself.

Does this have anything to do with the power of natural substances versus artificial laboratory-made products? It's tempting
to say yes. It's tempting to say that, although scientists can faithfully reproduce in the lab the exact chemical structure of a vita-

min, they cannot plug in the "essence of life"—that mystical quality that can be produced only in Mother Nature's laboratory. We can, in other words, build a man in every detail, right down to the DNA, but until we discover how to instill that as yet unknowable life force, our efforts will produce only a pile of immobile protoplasm.

While this argument is tempting, the facts argue against it. Scientists have been able to isolate sulforaphane, the phytochemical found in broccoli, and when they feed it to rats it has a greater protective effect against the development of cancer than does naturally occurring sulforaphane.

At present, when it comes to phytochemicals the sky's the limit as far as biochemists are concerned. There are seemingly countless phytochemicals, with estimates of thousands in tomatoes alone. The tremendous variety of phytochemicals raises the hope that if one type of phytochemical cannot stop cancer-causing agents from forming in the cell, another type will be able to pluck the agents out and get rid of them, or perhaps neutralize them after they are established.

Exciting stuff, huh? Stay tuned. More information is sure to follow in the media. In the meantime, the bottom line seems to suggest that Mom was right: take chicken soup for a cold, rather than a bottle of pills.

Exercise

Mini-Chapter 24

You Can't Run Away from Your Diet

There are many wonderful things we can say about exercise. And at this point in our history, it's likely that most Americans have heard them and can recite them by heart. The problem is that Americans know the benefits but refuse to participate. At present only about 8 percent of adults have said yes to regular, vigorous aerobic exercise. The rest have responded with an emphatic "no, thank you."

There are several reasons for the low response rate. First and foremost, the average American doesn't want to train like an athlete, and that's what vigorous aerobic exercise demands. Second, most feel they are too busy to squeeze in an hour of exercise, plus travel and prep time. Third, most find aerobic exercise boring and tedious. Fourth, all this effort doesn't produce anything other than fitness, and that's hard for our productivity-minded society to accept. We like to see tangible results for our efforts.

And fitness may bestow fewer benefits than thought. It is a myth that high levels of fitness are necessary for good health. In fact, once you have achieved at least an average level of fitness, you have essentially optimized the health benefits that fitness has to offer. The marathon runner, though more fit, isn't necessarily healthier than the gardener. And it's quite possible that the marathon runner is less healthy, if the gardener follows a better diet.

For proof, look at the many research studies conducted by the Institute for Aerobics Research in Dallas, Texas. All of their scientific studies support the following conclusions: If you are a couch potato, your health is in danger. If you exercise moderately each day, you reduce your risk of heart disease substantially.

There is very little additional health benefit to be derived from increasing your aerobic fitness beyond average levels.

It is the "process" of being active that is health-promoting. It is important to distinguish the process from the product (fitness), and we haven't done that until now. This is a welcome message, because it opens up a smorgasbord of opportunities. You can choose things to do that you like: gardening, volleyball, golf, walking through the park. Things you don't particularly like to do count too: cutting the grass, washing the car, painting, vacuuming, and dusting. All of these things count as effective, health-enhancing exercise.

It's likely that fitness experts will reject this notion because it's threatening to question something you have always held near and dear. It is especially difficult for fitness experts to accept the fact that megadoses of exercise can't counteract the health-destroying effects of a high-fat diet. Again, there is more than ample scientific proof from research studies demonstrating that people who run many miles each day may be in very poor health, primarily because of their diet. Clearly, you can't swim, row, cycle, or run away from your diet.

Mini-Chapter 25

Don't Put Yourself on the Spot

A variety of exercise gadgets promise to trim fat from the thighs or the waistline. You've seen the commercials on TV. All you have to do is purchase a scientifically designed gizmo for $39.95, place it between your knees, then squeeze your knees together fifty times each day. In no time, thigh fat will melt away. It's magic.

Attempting to rid fat from a particular area of the body (like the thighs) through specialized exercises is called spot reduction. The concept has been around a long time, and most people take for granted that it works. It doesn't. You cannot rid fat from a particular area of the body, no matter how specialized the exercise routine.

This is difficult for most of us to understand. Although it seems logical that the muscles beneath a layer of fat should be able to reach out and grab the surrounding fat and use it as fuel, things just don't work that way. The fat you use as fuel is mobilized from fat deposits throughout the body and dumped into the bloodstream. While you are doing sit-ups, for example, the fat you are using as fuel may be from your arms, neck, or calves.

For this reason, it is the total number of calories you burn during exercise that is important—not the location of the muscles doing the work. The more calories you burn, the more likely you are eventually to burn fat from the specific areas you want to reduce. Large muscle exercises such as walking are best because they burn the most calories per minute. By comparison, pumping out sit-ups involves only small muscles that burn relatively few calories. Moreover, small muscles are likely to fatigue quickly, well before you log any appreciable number of burned calories. To lose one pound of body fat, you must burn 3,500 calories. That's countless hours of horribly boring, and potentially damaging (to your lower back), sit-ups.

Your best bet is to gradually build up to walking several miles a day at a moderately brisk pace. A male adult will burn about 100 calories per mile, and a smaller female will burn about 80. When you get to the point where you are burning 300 to 500 calories per day, combined with a low-fat diet, you'll be right on course to get rid of the fatty areas you despise.

Though exercise is important, clearly the most important step you can take to reduce troublesome "love handles" or "saddlebags" is to follow the Jack Sprat low-fat diet. Deprive the fat stores of what they want most—dietary fat. Exercise will help and shouldn't be overlooked, but the effects of exercise to reduce body fatness pale in comparison with the effects of a low-fat diet.

Mini-Chapter 26

Fat-Burner Exercise

Fat-burning exercise is being promoted by health clubs and aerobics instructors. It's an approach that is supposed to help the body burn more fat during exercise. Is there anything to this, or is it much ado about nothing?

Like many of the principles we embrace in daily life, there is a small grain of truth attached to fat-burning exercise, but nothing more. Here's the grain of truth.

Dietary fat and carbohydrate are the two primary sources of fuel used by the body. Protein is used at times, but your body prefers to save protein for other duties. At rest, your body uses a mixture of approximately 60 percent fat and 40 percent carbohydrate. When you exercise, the mixture changes, progressively favoring carbohydrate as the work gets harder. And during maximum effort—dashing at top speed, for example—your body depends entirely on carbohydrate as fuel.

This means that the intensity of exercise is the determining factor in fuel mix. Herein lies the grain of truth. Because intensity governs fuel mix, it would appear that very low-intensity exercise should be the exercise of choice because the fuel mix would favor fat being burned as fuel. While this makes sense, there are many other factors that must be taken into consideration, including total calories expended. A comparison of low-intensity versus moderately high-intensity exercise may be helpful.

If you exercise for an hour at a low intensity (walking at 3.5 mph) you may expend approximately 300 calories. If your fuel mix was 50 percent fat and 50 percent carbohydrate, half the calories expended would come from fat, or 150 calories.

If you exercise for an hour at a moderately high intensity (jogging at 6 mph), you may expend approximately 700 calories. At the higher intensity, the fuel mix would slant toward carbohydrate and be on the order of 35 percent fat and 65 percent carbohydrate. Thus, 35 percent of the 700 calories would come from fat, or 245 calories.

These examples are oversimplifications of the physiological processes involved, and the numbers will vary from person to person. But the relationships are valid. And it is clearly demonstrated that a high percentage of fat in the fuel mix is only one piece of the puzzle.

What's more, there is no evidence to support the notion that burning a high percentage of fat or even a high amount of fat during exercise translates to a greater ultimate removal of fat from the body. This is because the metabolic pathways for carbohydrate and fat, and even protein, intertwine and overlap. The body can convert carbohydrate to fat, protein to fat, protein to carbohydrate, and so forth.

You should choose your exercise based on personal preference. Pick something that you enjoy, that is comfortable and convenient, and that you will do regularly. And reduce the need for fat burning by consuming less fat in the first place: it's a lot more effective than half-baked exercise schemes.

Mini-Chapter 27

From Gardening to Volleyball

Most people are surprised to learn that when it comes to exercise they have many more alternatives than they thought. If your goal is to look good, feel good, and be healthy, you can accomplish this by taking walks, working in the garden, participating in light sporting activities, and performing chores such as cutting the grass.

The key to effective exercise is to be physically active every day. Unless you need to prepare yourself for a difficult physical feat, like mountain hiking, you don't need to train like an athlete and you don't need to develop more than a moderate level of fitness. Beyond this moderate level, no additional health benefits accrue.

This approach differs greatly from the fitness dogma preached for the past thirty years. We now know that the old fitness dogma failed to make the distinction between exercising for the sake of producing physical fitness and exercising for health. At one time it was assumed that you had to train the same for both. Now we know better. And because we know better, this opens up a whole smorgasbord of exercise possibilities.

In the past, people believed that exercise had to produce a high level of fitness and that they were limited to such activities as jogging, swimming laps, rowing, and cross-country skiing. But since producing a high level of fitness is not a prerequisite for health, you can choose from among any and all physical activities that simply get you moving and keep you moving, whether they increase your fitness or not. The key to improved health is the "process" of being physically active. It is not fitness—the end "product" of physical activity.

But what about losing weight? Don't you need to bust a gut running around the football field in order to lose a few pounds? The answer is no. *A calorie is a calorie,* and it doesn't matter whether you expend that calorie running around a track with a grimace on your face or walking in the park, smiling ear to ear. The only thing your body knows is that the muscles are contracting, and they need energy. True, you will burn calories faster by running. But if you don't enjoy running, each minute you invest will seem like an hour. So why not spend a little extra time walking, knowing that the time will fly by because you are enjoying yourself?

There may be situations where exercise options are limited. For example, people with arthritis need exercise that avoids putting weight on joints, and being in the water is perfect. Similarly, people who suffer from exercise-induced asthma breathe better while active in the water than they do while active on land. The humidity from the water might have a beneficial effect on the respiratory system.

But even if you have to exercise in the water, this doesn't mean that you have to swim laps. On the contrary, opportunities abound. Watch people who go to swimming pools on hot summer days.

They get in the water and they walk, pushing their arms and legs against the resistance of the water. They play catch with a ball. They dive. They move every which way. They are having fun and exercising at the same time. Admittedly, swimming laps will give you more fitness. But you need to consider whether the tedium makes it a good choice for you.

The same thing goes for those who frequent gyms and health clubs. If you watch people on their first visit, they usually have fun trying out the variety of exercise equipment. They spend a few minutes on the treadmill, then switch over to the high-tech stationary cycle for a few more minutes, then to the stair climber and on to the muscle-building machines. They don't do a lot at each station, but overall their efforts add up to an hour of good exercise.

Unfortunately, all this changes when the professionals enter the picture and impose a workout schedule. Now, instead of spontaneously moving about the gym and enjoying the experience, you labor under the tyranny of a fitness-producing workout. Soon, you find that you no longer look forward to going to the gym, and eventually you find too many excuses to go back. And for good reason. Why would anyone want to work on their job for eight to ten hours, then finish off the day by going to the gym for a tedious workout? Only the most dedicated are capable of sustaining this kind of regimen. The rest of us crumble under the weight.

The best exercise advice we can give is, lighten up. If you're interested in producing a high level of fitness, you must train like an athlete. If being healthy, looking good, and feeling good are your goals, it's a lot easier than you think. Just get busy—and don't forget to have fun and enjoy it.

Mini-Chapter 28

24 Hours a Day

When you think of exercise as an aid to losing weight you probably think of aerobic exercise, and for good reason. Walking and other forms of aerobic exercise burn lots of calories each minute, and the more calories you burn each day the better your chances of losing body fat.

Most people discount the value of resistance exercises such as weight training, because weight training burns far fewer calories than aerobic exercise. By its nature, weight training involves spurts of activity followed by lengthy rest periods. An hour of weight training may involve only 20 minutes of actual exercise and 40 minutes of rest. Not a good formula for weight reduction.

But there is an aspect of weight training that has been overlooked when it comes to weight control. Because weight training adds muscle mass to the body, it may be the body's best friend when it comes to reducing body fat. Here's why.

The most prevalent tissue in the body is muscle—unless, of course, you are obese, in which case the most prevalent tissue would be fat. Muscle is metabolically active, whereas fat is virtually inert. Since muscle is the major tissue in the body and since it is metabolically active, you can see that your muscle mass is the major determinant of the amount of energy you expend each day. The more muscle mass you have, the more calories you will burn, and vice versa.

Adding a little muscle mass as a result of weight training can pay big dividends. This is because of the boost in the body's metabolism. Here's how it works.

If we assume that the average person burns about 1 calorie (kcal) per minute at rest, this adds up to 1,440 calories per day. A larger person would burn more, a smaller person would burn less. If this average person were to begin a weight training program and add muscle mass to his or her frame, it's possible that the metabolic rate would increase slightly.

But is a slight increase worth the effort? You bet. An increase in resting metabolism from 1 calorie per minute to 1.1 calorie would burn an additional 144 calories per day. That's the amount of energy required to walk nearly 2 miles. As you can see, a tiny boost in metabolism brought about by an increase in muscle mass pays dividends 24 hours a day.

This wonderful calorie-burning effect is available to women as well as men. But men have an advantage. Because of testosterone, men will add muscle mass to their bodies more quickly and easily than women. But women tend to be smaller and tend to burn fewer calories to begin with, and so even a very small change in a woman's metabolism will exert proportionally the same effect as a larger effect in a man.

But is it reasonable to expect American adults to embark upon a program of pumping iron? Unfortunately, no. We're simply too busy, too lazy, too uninspired, too . . . (you fill in the blank). But we're not too busy to build a little resistance exercise into our daily lives, and although a little effort won't be enough to build a lot of extra muscle, it will be sufficient to help you hold on to what you've got.

Holding on to what you've got is critical, especially in old age, because as you age you naturally lose muscle mass. The gradual loss of muscle mass contributes to a reduction in resting metabolic rate, which in turn contributes to the accumulation of unwanted body fat. This is called creeping obesity. By incorporating some resistance exercise into your daily life, you can slow down the loss of muscle and the complications associated with it.

Simple things such as climbing stairs and pressing (pushing to arm's length overhead) a filled milk carton overhead are examples of incorporating resistance exercise into daily life. If you don't do these kinds of things, the loss of muscle mass accelerates, and a vicious cycle begins.

First, there is the loss of muscle mass that leads to a loss of strength. Between age 50 and age 65, there is approximately a 20 percent loss of strength. After that, strength loss accelerates, and by age 75 you are about half as strong as you were as a young adult.

Next, because you lose strength, everyday tasks become more difficult. Since they are more difficult, you try to avoid them. Doing less leads to a further decline of muscle mass and strength, and it makes such tasks even more difficult. Climbing stairs is a perfect example. When people get old they sell their two-story home and buy a one-floor ranch. They don't want to have to struggle up the stairs. Living on one floor removes the challenge, but it also removes the stimulation stair climbing had on the leg muscles. Without such stimulation, the leg muscles lose mass and strength. In time, the muscles become so small and weak that climbing stairs is no longer an option.

Fortunately, there is evidence that even in old age you can reclaim some strength and muscle mass. Research has shown that people in their nineties doubled their muscle strength in only eight weeks by doing leg exercises; they were able to rise from sitting and walk more easily than they had in years. In addition, most were able to be less dependent on their canes and walkers.

The way to retain strength and muscle mass is to sustain a daily schedule of doing the kinds of things that are required in everyday life. Pushing yourself out of a chair, sitting, then pushing again and again is an example. Others include climbing stairs, lifting and carrying moderately heavy packages, pressing canned goods overhead and onto a shelf, and so forth. If you commit to doing something every day, no matter how little, you will make progress. But don't expect dramatic changes, and don't push yourself. Be comfortable in what you do, and never push to the point that you are out of breath or you risk injury.

This doesn't mean that you can't be more adventuresome and invest some effort into real weight training. On the contrary, feel free to join a gym or purchase some home equipment and go for it. But first, check with your doctor to make sure your body is up to the challenge.

References

Acheson, K.J., J.P. Flatt, and E. Jequier. "Glycogen Synthesis Versus Lipogenesis after a 500-Gram Carbohydrate Meal in Man." *Metabolism* 31 (1982): 1234-40.

Acheson, K.J., Y. Schutz, T. Bessard, et al. "Nutritional Influences on Lipogenesis and Thermogenesis after a Carbohydrate Meal." *American Journal of Physiology* 246, no. 9 (1984): E62-E70.

Adams, C.E., and K.J. Morgan. "Periodicity of Eating: Implications for Human Food Consumption." *Nutrition Research* 1 (1981): 525-50.

Ailhaud, G., et al. "Growth and Differentiation of Regional Adipose Tissue; Molecular and Hormonal Mechanisms." *International Journal of Obesity* 2 (1991): 87.

American College of Sports Medicine. "Position Statement on Proper and Improper Weight Loss Programs." *Medicine and Science in Sports and Exercise* 15, no. 1 (1983): ix.

American Dietetic Association. "Position of the American Dietetic Association: Health Implication of Dietary Fiber." *Journal of the American Dietetic Association* 8 (1988): 216.

American Dietetic Association. "Position of the American Dietetic Association: Optimal Weight as a Health Promotion Strategy." *Journal of the American Dietetic Association* 89 (1989): 1814-17.

American Dietetic Association. "Position of the American Dietetic Association: Vegetarian Diets—Technical Support Paper." *Journal of the American Dietetic Association* 88 (1988): 352-54.

American Dietetic Association. "Position of the American Dietetic Association: Very-Low-Calorie Weight Loss Diets." *Journal of the American Dietetic Association* 90 (1990): 722-26.

American Heart Association. "Heart and Stroke Facts." National Center, Dallas, Texas, 1994.

American Heart Association. "Dietary Guidelines for Healthy American Adults. A Statement for Physicians and Health Professions by the Nutrition Committee, American Heart Association." *Circulation* 77 (1988): 721A-724A.

American Institute of Cancer Research. "Research Update: AICR Study Finds Vegetable Compound Effective against Cancer." *AICR Newsletter* 27 (Spring 1990): 12.

American Medical Association, Council on Scientific Affairs. "Dietary Fiber and Health." *Journal of the American Medical Association* 262 (1989): 542-46.

Anderson, J., et al. "Dietary Fiber and Diabetes: A Comprehensive Review and Practical Application." *Journal of the American Dietetic Association* 87 (1987): 1189-97.

"Another Slap in the Face for Saturated Fat." *Men's Health Newsletter,* January 1989, 3.

Atkinson, R.L., and F.X. Pi-Sunyer. "Very-Low-Calorie Diets." *American Journal of Clinical Nutrition* 56 (1992): 175S.

Ballor, D.L., et al. "Resistance Weight Training during Caloric Restriction Enhances Lean Body Weight Maintenance." *American Journal of Clinical Nutrition* 47 (1988): 19.

Ballor, D.L., and R.E. Keesey. "A Meta-Analysis of the Factors Affecting Exercise-Induced Changes in Body Mass, Fat Mass and Fat-Free Mass in Males and Females." *International Journal of Obesity* 15 (1991): 71.

Baumgartner, R.N. "Bioelectric Impedance for Body Composition." In *Exercise and Sport Sciences Reviews,* vol. 18, edited by K.B. Pandolf and J.O. Holloszy. Baltimore: Williams and Wilkins, 1990.

Berry, E.M., J. Hirsch, J. Most, et al. "The Role of Dietary Fat in Human Obesity." *International Journal of Obesity* 10 (1986): 123-31.

Bjorntorp, P. "Adipose Tissue Distribution and Function." *International Journal of Obesity* 15 (1991): 67.

Blackburn, G.L., et al. "Weight Cycling: The Experience of Human Dieters." *American Journal of Clinical Nutrition* 49 (1989): 1105.

Blair, S.N., H.W. Kohl, R.S. Paffenbarger, et al. "Physical Fitness and All-Cause Mortality: A Prospective Study of Healthy Men and Women." *Journal of the American Medical Association* 262 (1989): 2395-401.

Block, G. "Vitamin C and Cancer Prevention: The Epidemiologic Evidence." *American Journal of Clinical Nutrition* 53 (1991): 270S-82S.

Bray, G.A. "Lipogenesis in Human Adipose Tissue: Some Effects of Nibbling and Gorging." *Journal of Clinical Investigation* 51 (1972): 537-48.

Brody, J. *Jane Brody's Nutrition Book.* New York: Norton, 1981.

Brooks, C. "Adult Participation in Physical Activities Requiring Moderate to High Levels of Energy Expenditure." *Physician and Sportsmedicine* 15, no. 4 (1987): 119-32.

———. "Adult Physical Activity Behavior: A Trend Analysis." *Journal of Clinical Epidemiology* 41, no. 4 (1988): 385-92.

Burgess, N., et al. "Effects of Very Low Calorie Diets on Body Composition and Resting Metabolic Rate in Obese Men and Women." *Journal American Dietetic Association* 91 (1991): 430.

Burton, G.W., M.G. Traber. "Vitamin E: Antioxidant Activity, Biokinetics, and Bioavailability." *Annual Review of Nutrition* 10 (1990): 357-82.

Campaigne, B. "Body Fat Distribution in Females: Metabolic Consequences and Implications for Weight Loss." *Medicine and Science in Sports and Exercise* 22 (1990): 291.

Caspersen, C., and R.A. Pollard. "Prevalence of Physical Activity in the United States and Its Relationship to Disease Risk Factors." *Medicine and Science in Sports and Exercise* 19, no. 2: (1987) S6.

Clark, N. "How to Pack a Meatless Diet Full of Nutrients." *Physician and Sportsmedicine* 19 (1991): 31-34.

Davies, P.S.W., et al. "The Distribution of Subcutaneous and Internal Fat in Man." *Annals of Human Biology* 13 (1986): 189.

Dietz, W.H., Jr., and S.L. Gortmaker. "Do We Fatten Our Children at the Television Set? Obesity and Television Viewing in Children and Adolescents." *Pediatrics* 75 (1985): 807-12.

Dishman, R. "Exercise Compliance: A New View for Public Health." *Physician and Sportsmedicine* 14 (1986): 127-45.

Drewnowski, A., J.D. Brunzell, K. Sande, et al. "Sweet Tooth Reconsidered: Taste Responsiveness in Human Obesity." *Physiology and Behavior* 35 (1985): 617-22.

Dudley, G. "Metabolic Consequences of Resistive-Type Exercise." *Medicine and Science in Sports and Exercise* 20 (1988): S158-S161.

Dullo, A.G., and L. Girardier. "Adaptive Changes in Energy Expenditure During Refeeding Following Low-Calorie Intake: Evidence for a Specific Metabolic Component Favoring Fat Storage." *American Journal of Clinical Nutrition* 52 (1990): 415.

Durenberg, P., et al. "Changes in Fat-Free Mass During Weight Loss Measured by Bioelectrical Impedance and by Densitometry." *American Journal of Clinical Nutrition* 49 (1989): 33.

Elliott, D.L., et al. "Sustained Depression of the Resting Metabolic Rate After Massive Weight Loss." *American Journal of Clinical Nutrition* 49 (1989): 93.

Enos, W.F., R.H. Holmes, and J. Beyer. "Coronary Disease Among United States Soldiers Killed in Korea." *Journal of American Medical Association* 152 (1953): 1090-93.

Fabry, P., J. Fodor, A. Hejl, et al. "The Frequency of Meals: Its Relation to Overweight, Hypercholesterolemia, and Decreased Glucose-Tolerance." *Lancet* 2 (1964): 614-15.

Forbes, G.B., et al. "Is Bioimpedance a Good Predictor of Body Composition Change?" *American Journal of Clinical Nutrition* 56 (1992): 4.

Fowler, B.A., et al. "Total and Subcutaneous Adipose Tissue in Women: The Measurement of Distribution and Accurate Prediction of Quantity by Using Magnetic Resonance Imaging." *American Journal of Clinical Nutrition* 54 (1991): 18.

Frontera, W.R., et al. "Strength Conditioning in Older Men: Skeletal Muscle Hypertrophy and Improved Function." *Journal of Applied Physiology* 64 (1988): 1038.

References

Gentry, M. "Free Radicals: What Are They, and How Do They Affect Your Health?" *American Institute for Cancer Research Newsletter* 28 (1990): 7.

"Green Light for Splurging." *Men's Health Newsletter,* September 1989, 8.

Griffin, G.C., and W.P. Castelli. "All About Your Cholesterol Numbers." *Prevention,* March 1989, 55-59.

Heyward, V.H. "Predictive Accuracy of Three Field Methods for Estimating Relative Body Fatness of Nonobese and Obese Women." *International Journal of Sports Nutrition* 2 (1992): 75.

Hirsch, J., et al. "The Fat Cell." *Medical Clinics of North America* 73 (1989): 83-96.

Hodgetts, V., et al. "Factors Controlling Fat Mobilization from Human Subcutaneous Adipose During Exercise." *Journal of Applied Physiology* 71 (1991): 445.

Horwitt, M. "Data Supporting Supplementation of Humans with Vitamin E." *Journal of Nutrition* 121 (1991): 424-29.

International Collaborative Group. "Circulating Cholesterol Level and Risk of Death from Cancer in Men Aged 40-69 Years—Experience of International Collaborative Group." *Journal of American Medical Association* 248 (1982): 2853-59.

Johnston, F.E. "Body Fat Deposition in Adult Obese Women. I. Patterns of Fat Distribution." *American Journal of Clinical Nutrition* 47 (1988): 225.

Kaplan, N.M., and J. Stamler. Prevention of Coronary Heart Disease: Practical Management of the Risk Factors. Philadelphia: Saunders, 1983.

Katahn, M. *The T-Factor Diet.* New York: Norton, 1989.

Katch, F.I., P.M. Clarkson, W. Kroll, et al. "Effects of Sit Up Exercise Training on Adipose Cell Size and Adiposity." *Research Quarterly for Exercise and Sport* 55 (1984): 242-47.

Kendler, B. "Vegetarianism: Nutritional Aspects and Implications for Health Professionals." *Journal of Holistic Medicine* 6 (1984): 161-70.

Kessey, R.E. "A Set-Point Theory of Obesity." In *Handbook of Eating Disorders,* edited by K.D. Brownell and J.P. Foreyt. New York: Basic Books, 1986.

Kowalski, R.E. *The 8-Week Cholesterol Cure.* New York: Harper and Row, 1987.

Lanska, D. "A Prospective Study on Body Fat Distribution and Weight Loss." *International Journal of Obesity* 9 (1985): 241.

LaPorte, R., and D. LaPorte. "A New Look at Exercise and Fitness." *Executive Health Report* 24, no. 12 (1988): 1-2.

LaPorte, R.E., S. Dearwater, J.A. Cauley, et al. "Physical Activity or Cardiovascular Fitness: Which Is More Important for Health?" *Physician and Sportsmedicine* 13 (1985): 145-50.

Lissner, L., D.A. Levitsky, B.J. Strupp, et al. "Dietary Fat and the Regulation of Energy Intake in Human Subjects." *American Journal of Clinical Nutrition* 46 (1987): 886-92.

McNamara, J.J., M.A. Molot, J.F. Stremple, et al. "Coronary Artery Disease in Combat Casualties in Vietnam." *Journal of American Medical Association* 216 (1971): 1185-87.

Meydani, S.N., et al. "Vitamin E Supplementation Enhances Cell-Mediated Immunity in Healthy Elderly Subjects." *American Journal of Clinical Nutrition* 52 (1990): 557-63.

Moncada, S., and J.R. Vance. "Arachidonic Acid Metabolites and the Interactions Between Platelets and Blood-Vessel Walls." *New England Journal of Medicine* 300 (1979): 1142-47.

National Institutes of Health Consensus Development Conference. "Lowering Blood Cholesterol to Prevent Heart Disease." *Journal of the American Medical Association* 253 (1985): 2080.

Olsen, E. "Putting Fun Back in Fitness." *Reader's Digest,* August 1988, 145-50.

Ostlund, R.E., et al. "The Ratio of Waist-to-Hip Circumference, Plasma Insulin Level, and Glucose Intolerance as Independent Predictors of the HDL2 Cholesterol Level in Older Adults." *New England Journal of Medicine* 332 (1990): 229.

Packer, L. "Protective Role of Vitamin E in Biological Systems." *American Journal of Clinical Nutrition* 53 (1991): 1050S-1055S.

References

Paffenbarger, R.S., Jr., A.L. Wing, R.T. Hyde. "Physical Activity as an Index of Heart Attack Risk in College Alumni." *American Journal of Epidemiology* 108 (1978): 161-75.

Pritikin, N. *The Pritikin Program for Diet and Exercise.* New York: Grosset and Dunlap, 1979.

Pyorala, K. "Dietary Cholesterol in Relation to Plasma Cholesterol and Coronary Heart Disease." *American Journal Clinical Nutrition* 45 (1987): 1176.

Rebuffe-Scrive, M. "Fat Cell Metabolism in Different Regions in Women: The Effect of the Menstrual Cycle, Pregnancy, and Lactation." *Journal of Clinical Investigation* 75 (1985): 1973.

Rodin, J., et al. "Weight Cycling and Fat Distribution." *International Journal of Obesity* 14 (1990): 303.

Rouse, I.L., L.J. Beilin, B.K. Armstrong, et al. "Blood-Pressure-Lowering Effect of a Vegetarian Diet: Controlled Trial in Normotensive Subjects." *Lancet* 8 (1983): 5-10.

Sacks, F.M., B. Rosner, and E.H. Kass. "Blood Pressure in Vegetarians." *American Journal of Epidemiology* 100 (1974): 390-98.

Schelkun, P.H. "Treating Overweight Patients: Don't Weigh Success in Pounds." *Physician and Sportsmedicine* 21, no. 2 (1993): 148.

Sedlick, D., and B. Cohen. "The Effect of Acute Nutritional Status on Postexercise Energy Expenditure." *Medicine and Science in Sports and Exercise* 22 (1990): S49.

Shimokatam, H., et al. "Studies in the Distribution of Body Fat: The Effect of Age, Sex, and Obesity." *Journal Gerontology* 44 (1989): 66.

Sims, E.A.H., and E. Danforth. "Expenditure and Storage of Energy in Man." *Journal of Clinical Investigation* 79 (1987): 1019-25.

Smith, S. " 'Trans' Fatty Acids in Processed Foods . . . Something to Worry About?" *Environmental Nutrition* 11 (1988): 6-7.

Stamford, B. "Apples and Pears." *Physician and Sportsmedicine* 19 (1991): 123-24.

―――. "Exercise and the Elderly." In *Exercise and Sport Sciences Reviews,* vol. 16, edited by K.B. Pandolf. New York: Macmillan, 1988.

————. "Meals and Timing of Exercise." *Physician and Sportsmedicine* 17 (1989): 151.

————. "What Cholesterol Means to You." *Physician and Sportsmedicine* 18 (1990): 149.

————. "What Is Cellulite?" *Physician and Sportsmedicine* 14 (1986): 226.

Stamford, B.A., S. Matter, R.D. Fell, et al. "Effects of Smoking Cessation on Weight Gain, Metabolic Rate, Caloric Consumption and Blood Lipids." *American Journal of Clinical Nutrition* 43 (1986): 486-94.

Stamford, B., and P. Shimer. *Fitness Without Exercise.* New York: Warner, 1990.

Steinberg, D., J. Witztum. "Lipoproteins and Atherogenesis." *Journal of the American Medical Association* 264 (1990): 3047-52.

Thompson, P.D., E.M. Cullinane, S.P. Sady, et al. "Modest Changes in High-Density Lipoprotein Concentration and Metabolism with Prolonged Exercise Training." *Circulation* 78, no. 1 (1988): 25-34.

Tonkelaer, I., et al. "Factors Influencing Waist/Hip Ratio in Randomly Selected Pre-and Post-menopausal Women." *International Journal of Obesity* 13 (1989): 817.

Tremblay, A., et al. "Impact of Dietary Fat Content and Fat Oxidation on Energy Intake in Humans." *American Journal of Clinical Nutrition* 49 (1989): 799.

Vogel, J.A., and M.J. Kasper. "Body Fat Assessment in Women: Special Considerations." *Sports Medicine* 13 (1992): 245.

Walker, J., L.C. Collins, L. Nannini, and B.A. Stamford. "Potentiating Effects of Cigarette Smoking and Moderate Exercise on the Thermic Effect of a Meal." *International Journal of Obesity* 16 (1992): 341-47.

Waller, B.F. "Exercise-Related Sudden Death." *Postgraduate Medicine* 83, no. 8 (1988): 273-82.

————. "Exercise-Related Sudden Death in Young (Age <30 Years) and Old (Age >30 Years) Conditioned Subjects." *Cardiovascular Clinics* 15, no. 2 (1985): 9-73.

————. "Sudden Death in Middle-aged Conditioned Subjects; Coronary Atherosclerosis Is the Culprit." *Mayo Clinic Proceedings* 62, no. 7 (1987): 634-36.

Waller, B.F., and W.C. Roberts. "Sudden Death While Running in Conditioned Runners Aged 40 Years or Over." *American Journal of Cardiology* 45, no. 6 (1980): 1292-300.

Waterhouse, D. *Outsmarting the Female Fat Cell.* New York: Hyperion, 1993.

Wellness Encyclopedia. University of California, Berkeley. Boston: Houghton Mifflin, 1991.

Whitney, E.N., and S.R. Rolfes. *Understanding Nutrition,* 6th ed. St. Paul: West Publishing, 1993.

Wing, R., et al. "Change In Waist-Hip Ratio with Weight Loss and Its Association with Change in Cardiovascular Risk Factors." *American Journal of Clinical Nutrition* 55 (1992): 1086.

Yamanada, W. "Vitamins and Cancer Prevention: How Much Do We Know?" *Postgraduate Medicine* 82 (1987): 149-51.

Index

adipose tissue, 230, 241. *See also* fat cells
aerobics, 49, 51, 295. *See also* exercise
afterburn, 4, 50-52. *See also exercise*
alcohol, 240, 279-80
American Cancer Society, 27, 244
American Diabetes Association, 27
American Dietetic Association, 70, 270, 303
American Heart Association, 26, 244, 303-4
aminophylline, 229. *See also* spot reduction; thigh cream
anemia, 269
antioxidants, 5, 271-74. *See also* atherosclerosis; free radicals; minerals; vitamins
arteries, 274. *See also* atherosclerosis; blood vacuuming
atherosclerosis, 28-30, 53, 274. *See also* blood clots; free radicals; heart attacks; HDL; LDL; serum cholesterol

badminton, 47. *See also* exercise
banjo string belly, 225
bee pollen, 271. *See also* supplements
beef, 22; ground, 35-37, 261; ground beef products, 36, 261; tallow, 33-34
bile, 267
blood, 25, 31; bloodstream, 25, 31, 50-51, 53, 223, 226, 239, 257, 267, 293; clotting of, 52-53, 274; sugar, 78, 257-58; tests of,

33; vacuuming of, 53; volume of, 239
blood pressure, 1, 4, 6, 22, 32, 37, 78, 226; effects of salt on, 281. *See also* hypertension
body fat: caloric content of, 14, 294; metabolism of, 15, 24, 255, 301; reduction of, 17-18, 28, 48, 228, 258, 300; stores of, 17, 223; in Americans, 23; buttocks and, 24, 225-26, 228, 230, 233, 238; and fat cells, 25, 241; caloric balance and, 59; health risks of, 225; abdominal fat, 226-27; of women, 228; essential, 234; measurement of, 236-37; brown fat, 251; effects of insulin on, 257; alcohol and, 279
bones, 234, 261-63, 270. *See also* calcium; exercise; osteoporosis
breast-feeding, 230, 242

calcium, 73, 259, 262, 269-70. *See also* minerals; osteoporosis; supplements
cancer: of breast, 27, 244-45; of colon, 70, 267; of prostate, 245. *See also* estradiol; estrogen; hormones
constipation, 70, 267. *See also* fiber; hemorrhoids; colon cancer
controlled cheating, 2, 5, 41
cholesterol: dietary, 31, 283-85; dietary, and children, 22, 241-42; serum, 4, 11, 31, 33-34, 262; HDL, 12, 274; LDL, 31, 274; production of, by body,

milk: changing from whole to skim, 4; as major source of dietary fat, 21-22, 36-38, 261; source of calcium, 73; important source of fat for babies and infants, 241-42
minerals: RDA on Jack Sprat plan, 70; inadequate intake on low calorie diets, 73; animal versus vegetable sources, 269; as antioxidants, 271; advisability of taking more than the RDA of, 275
monounsaturated fat, 31-32. *See also* fat
More Smart Choices, 215-18
muscles: glycogen stored in, 24; post-meal blood flow and, 50-51; sustaining of, 61; breakdown when dieting, 224-25; protein and, 261; calorie burning and, 293; loss in aging, 301-2
M&M's, 10, 42

National Cancer Institute, 245
Nutrasweet, 17

oat bran, 33, 69, 267
oatmeal, 12, 33, 258
obesity: in early life, 22, 242; creeping, 235, 301; and flim-flam weight loss schemes, 247; and chemical imbalance, 249; and genetic abnormalities, 249; and brown fat, 251-52; impact of sugar on, 257; and fake fat and fake sugar, 265; fiber and, 266
obesity patterns: android, 225; gynoid, 225
oils, 33-34
Ornish, Dean, 29

osteoporosis, 262, 270. *See also* bones; calcium; exercise
oxygen, 53
overeating, 241

pancreas, 25. *See also* diabetes; insulin
pasta, 71, 258, *See also* carbohydrates
Pauling, Linus, 272-74
phytochemicals, 286-87
Pillsbury Dough Boy, 241
polyunsaturated fat, 30-33. *See also* essential dietary fat
popcorn, 72, 282
potassium, 237, 239, 259. *See also* minerals; supplements
Power of the Lean, 1
premenstrual syndrome, 280. *See also* hormones
pretzels, 77, 282
protein: and pizza, 10; in muscle, 16; consumption of, 29, 61, 2 250; as dietary staple, 261-64; vegetarianism and, 269; egg whites and, 284; as fuel, 295-96
puberty, 234, 245
public relations team, 20

quick fixes, 17, 231

ratio (total cholesterol/HDL), 12
resistance exercise, 300-301. *See also* muscles
rice bran, 267
roughage, 266. *See also* fiber
rowing, 46-47, 297. *See also* exercise; fitness
running, 12-13, 49, 228, 298. *See also* exercise; fitness; jogging; marathon running